O A E L
OXFORD AMERICAN ENDOCRINOLOGY LIBRARY

Obesity and Type 2 Diabetes Mellitus

O A E L

OXFORD AMERICAN ENDOCRINOLOGY LIBRARY

Obesity and Type 2 Diabetes Mellitus

John P. Sheehan, MD, FACE, FACN

Medical Director
North Coast Institute of Diabetes and Endocrinology, Inc. and
Associate Clinical Professor of Medicine
Case Western Reserve University
Cleveland, Ohio

Margaret M. Ulchaker, MSN, RN, CDE, CNP, NP-C, BC-ADM

Endocrine Nurse Practitioner
North Coast Institute of Diabetes and Endocrinology, Inc. and
Clinical Instructor
Frances Payne Bolton School of Nursing
Case Western Reserve University
Cleveland, Ohio

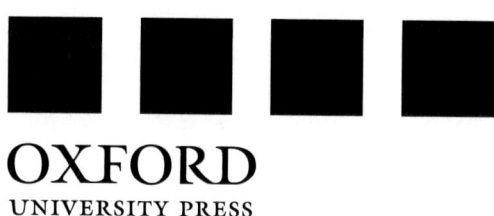

OXFORD
UNIVERSITY PRESS

OXFORD

UNIVERSITY PRESS

Oxford University Press, Inc., publishes works that further
Oxford University's objective of excellence
in research, scholarship, and education.

Oxford New York

Auckland Cape Town Dar es Salaam Hong Kong Karachi
Kuala Lumpur Madrid Melbourne Mexico City Nairobi
New Delhi Shanghai Taipei Toronto

With offices in

Argentina Austria Brazil Chile Czech Republic France Greece
Guatemala Hungary Italy Japan Poland Portugal Singapore
South Korea Switzerland Thailand Turkey Ukraine Vietnam

Copyright © 2012 by Oxford University Press, Inc.

Published by Oxford University Press, Inc.
198 Madison Avenue, New York, New York 10016
www.oup.com

Library of Congress Cataloging-in-Publication Data

Sheehan, John,
Obesity and type 2 diabetes mellitus / John P. Sheehan, Margaret M. Ulchaker.
p. ; cm. — (Oxford American endocrinology library)
Obesity and type two diabetes mellitus
Includes bibliographical references.
ISBN 978-0-19-974021-5 (pbk. : alk. paper)
I. Ulchaker, Margaret M.   II. Title.   III. Title: Obesity and type two diabetes
mellitus.   IV. Series: Oxford American endocrinology library.
[DNLM: 1. Diabetes Mellitus, Type 2.   2. Comorbidity.   3. Obesity. WK 810]
LC-classification not assigned
616.4'62–dc23   2011028750

9 8 7 6 5 4 3 2 1
Printed in the United States of America
on acid-free paper

Disclosures

Dr. Sheehan has been a consultant and promotional speaker for Amylin, Lilly, Novo Nordisk, Sanofi-Aventis, and GSK, as well as a promotional speaker for Merck.

Dedication

I dedicate this book to my wife, Pauline Mary, whose diagnosis with diabetes after our marriage during my histopathology residency program caused me to change my career path to endocrinology in a quest to find the best management options to prevent complications.

Contents

Preface

We are in the midst of a global epidemic of type 2 diabetes mellitus (T2DM) and obesity, with escalating health care costs related to the burden of complications. Obesity is intertwined with T2DM both in terms of increasing the risk of development of T2DM and in magnifying the associated morbidity and premature mortality. In this book, we provide a current, up-to-date, concise review of diagnostic criteria and pathophysiology of T2DM and obesity, with an aim to guide the reader from the point of diagnosis through the multitude of new treatment options, and then through the surveillance and management of complications and special situations.

Optimal care for the individual with T2DM requires not only commitment of the individual but also the involvement of a dedicated health care team. We each have family members afflicted with diabetes mellitus, so the quest for control to minimize complications is not only professional but also personal. We have a combined experience of over 50 years in the field of endocrinology and have worked as a team for 25 years both in the university-based setting and the private-practice setting, bringing a unique blend of background, education, and experience.

Introduction

Obesity and type 2 diabetes mellitus (T2DM) frequently coexist, with approximately 90% of T2DM patients being obese. The global epidemic of obesity is also heralding an epidemic of T2DM, which is being diagnosed earlier in life and is becoming a major burden on the health care system. In 2007, the annual cost of diabetes in the United States was $174 billion, and T2DM accounts for one in every ten health care dollars spent. When pre-diabetes is added, the cost soars to $218 billion.[1] Clinical trials have shown that T2DM can be prevented/delayed and that microvascular and macrovascular complications can be minimized/prevented. The medical costs associated with obesity have risen to an estimated $147 billion.[2] T2DM is a coronary risk equivalent. This implies that the risk of a first myocardial infarction (MI) in an individual with T2DM is equivalent to that of a second MI in a non-diabetic individual: the 7-year incidence is approximately 20%.[3] Since individuals with a prior MI are referred for cardiac rehabilitation, this emphasizes the need for urgent attention to risk factor modification for all individuals with T2DM.

References

1. Dall TM, Zhang Y, Chen Y et al. The economic burden of diabetes. *Health Affairs*. 2010;29(2):297–303.

2. Finkelstein EA, Trogdon JC, Cohen JW, et al. Annual medical spending attributable to obesity: payer- and service-specific estimates. *Health Affairs*. 2009;28(5): w822–831. Available at: http://diabetes.niddk.nih.gov/dm/pubs/statistics/.

3. Haffner SM, Lehto S, Ronnemaa T, et al. Mortality from coronary heart disease in subjects with type 2 diabetes and in nondiabetic subjects with and without prior myocardial infarction. *N Engl J Med*. 1998;339(4):229–234.

Chapter 1

Epidemiology, Populations at Risk, and Health/ Socioeconomic Impact

Epidemiology

T2DM

The prevalence of T2DM is escalating dramatically. In those 20 years of age and above, DM involves approximately 11.3% of the population in the United States. It is estimated that 35% of the population aged 20 or older is in the pre-diabetes stage of the disease.[1] Pre-diabetes is defined as either impaired fasting glucose (IFG) (fasting plasma glucose [FPG] 100–125 mg/dL) or impaired glucose tolerance (IGT) (2-hour postprandial plasma glucose (PPG) 140–199 mg/dL). Patients may have isolated IFG, isolated IGT with normal FPG, or both IFG and IGT. Isolated IFG tends to carry a lower risk of future progression to overt T2DM and carries with it a lower macrovascular risk.

The prevalence of T2DM is especially high in minority populations, who for multiple reasons tend to have worse glycemic control and a greater propensity for diabetic complications. A multitude of factors affect the development of T2DM and the subsequent seeking of health care. Issues include acculturation, health beliefs, dietary preferences, fears, use of alternative medicines, socioeconomic status, religious beliefs, health literacy, and cultural competence of the health care provider. The emergence of ethnically focused, culturally sensitive diabetes clinics holds great promise to reduce the burden of complications in these populations.[2]

Obesity

The prevalence of obesity continues to rise dramatically across the world. Recent prevalence data in the United States are listed in Table 1.1.

Table 1.1 U.S. Population by Weight	
BMI	% of Population 20 Years of Age and Older
<25	31.6%
≥25	68%
≥30	33.8%
≥40	5.7 %

Overall, more than 68% of the U.S. population is either overweight or obese, with the highest prevalence being in minority females. Childhood obesity is of particular concern, given the ramifications of obesity-related illnesses. Approximately 12.4% of children aged 2 to 5 are overweight, increasing to 17% of children aged 6 to 11 and 17.6% of children aged 12 to 19.[3] The prevalence of childhood obesity is such that many have predicted that it will lead to reduced life expectancy for current children for the first time in over a century.

Metabolic Syndrome

The prevalence of the metabolic syndrome is on the rise—not unexpectedly, given the associations with obesity and glucose intolerance. The most recent estimate for the prevalence of the metabolic syndrome is approximately 25% of the general U.S. population, with the prevalence increasing dramatically with advancing age. The prevalence of the metabolic syndrome is also higher in minority populations, with attendant risk of both T2DM and macrovascular disease.

Populations at Risk for T2DM

It is critical to diagnose T2DM as early as possible with a view to optimizing glycemic control and preventing devastating microvascular and macrovascular complications. Therefore, screening is advocated for all individuals as follows:

1. Screening should begin at age 45 years.
2. Screen earlier those individuals who have a BMI ≥25 and additional risk factors:
   a. First-degree relative with diabetes
   b. Physical inactivity
   c. History of delivering a baby >9 lbs or a history of prior gestational diabetes mellitus (GDM). Women with GDM should be screened 6 to 12 weeks postpartum and periodically thereafter. In women with prior GDM, the higher the postpartum BMI, the earlier the onset of T2DM.
   d. HbA1c ≥5.7%
   e. History of IFG
   f. History of IGT
   g. Women with polycystic ovarian syndrome. There is a four- to five-fold lifetime increased risk of T2DM.
   h. Hypertension (HTN), defined as BP ≥140/90 mmHg or receiving treatment for HTN
   i. High-density lipoprotein cholesterol (HDL-C) level <35 mg/dL and/or triglyceride level >250 mg/dL
   j. Members of a high-risk ethnic population such as Latino, African American, Asian American, Native American, and Pacific Islander
   k. Presence of other conditions associated with insulin resistance, such as acanthosis nigricans or severe obesity
   l. Unexplained microvascular complications such as neuropathy that could be consistent with T2DM
   m. Elements of the metabolic syndrome

Caveat: If clinical suspicion is high and screening FPG or HbA1c is equivocal, always do a 2-hour glucose tolerance test.[4]

Health and Socioeconomic Impact

Obesity, metabolic syndrome, and T2DM all contribute significantly to health care costs via associated complications. Obesity-related illnesses include:

1. Degenerative joint disease
2. Cholelithiasis
3. Gout
4. Sleep apnea
5. Cancer (breast, colorectal, endometrial, and prostate)
6. Cardiovascular disease
7. T2DM
8. Hypertension
9. Dyslipidemia
10. Depression

T2DM is a very costly disorder, at an annual cost of $174 billion, with direct costs accounting for $116 billion and indirect costs accounting for $58 billion. Most of the direct costs are related to macrovascular disease management with associated costly hospitalizations.[1] Microvascular complication management is also costly, especially for end-stage renal disease (ESRD). In 2008, the costs for the Medicare ESRD program for individuals with diabetes were $10.57 billion.[5]

The indirect costs of T2DM are equally devastating and include:

1. Disability and inability to work
2. Loss of employment
3. Loss of income to family
4. Loss of tax revenue to society
5. Burden to family members
6. Burden to employers in terms of health care insurance premiums and days lost from work
7. Burden to the health care system
8. Burden to the government via Medicare and Medicaid

Obesity is associated with over 112,000 excess deaths due to cardiovascular disease and an increase in overall health care costs.[3]

The lifestyle and medication adherence elements of obesity, hypertension, dyslipidemia, and T2DM have brought about changes in employee health insurance premiums and deductibles. Many employers are increasing premiums and deductibles for individuals who do not meet BMI, HbA1c, blood pressure, and/or lipid goals and who continue smoking cigarettes. The results of this financially incentivized approach on behavior changes regarding obesity, hypertension, dyslipidemia, smoking cessation, and T2DM has yet to be determined.

References

1. U.S. Department of Health and Human Services, Centers for Disease Control and Prevention. *National Diabetes Fact Sheet: National Estimates and General Information on Diabetes and Prediabetes in the United States*, 2011. Atlanta, GA.

2. Cabellero AE. Type 2 diabetes in the Hispanic and Latino population: Challenges and opportunities. *Curr Opion Endocrinol Diabetes Obes.* 2007;14(2):151–57.

3. U.S. Department of Health and Human Services, National Institutes of Health, National Institute of Diabetes and Digestive and Kidney Disease. *Statistics Related to Overweight and Obesity.* NIH Publication Number 04-4158. February 2010.

4. American Diabetes Association. Standards of medical care in diabetes—2011. *Diabetes Care.* 2011;34(Suppl 1):S1–61.

5. USRDS 2009 Annual Data Report. Available at U.S. Renal Data System website, www.usrds.org/adr.htm. Accessed Feb. 28, 2011.

Chapter 2

Diagnostic Criteria

T2DM

T2DM may be diagnosed as follows:[1]

1. FPG ≥126 mg/dL on two occasions in an ambulatory setting
2. A casual 2-hour PPG ≥200 mg/dL on two occasions in an ambulatory setting
3. A 2-hour GTT conducted with a 75-g glucose load resulting in a 2-hour PPG ≥200 mg/dL
4. HbA1c ≥6.5%[1–3]

Approximately 10% of patients with T2DM over the age of 35 and 25% of patients with T2DM below that age actually have latent autoimmune diabetes of adulthood (LADA). Clues to the presence of LADA include:

1. BMI <30
2. The presence of other autoimmune diseases such as Hashimoto's thyroiditis, vitiligo, etc.
3. A low-normal C-peptide level
4. Positive glutamic acid decarboxylase-65 (GAD-65) antibodies

LADA patients tend to have a more gradual loss of beta-cell function than patients with conventional type 1 diabetes mellitus (T1DM). However, they will ultimately need full physiologic insulin replacement therapy, similar to the patient with T1DM.[4]

The diagnostic criteria for T2DM are based on the premise that an FPG ≥126 mg/dL in general predicts a 2-hr PPG ≥200 mg/dL, which in turn predicts retinopathy. Thus, T2DM diagnostic criteria are really targeting risk for the specific microvascular complication of retinopathy. However, other microvascular complications such as neuropathy may occur at lower ambient glucose levels, as does macrovascular disease. Overreliance on the FPG and HbA1c criteria can underdiagnose patients, especially in the geriatric years. In practice, a 2-hr 75-g post-glucose load GTT is helpful in this setting where suspicion of T2DM is high or where there is evidence of unexplained microvascular disease, such as neuropathy. In 2010, the now better-standardized HbA1c was added to the diagnostic testing. The HbA1c is convenient and reproducible and may be helpful, but may lead to underdiagnosis. Failure to diagnose T2DM at its true onset can be devastating: up to 50% of patients with T2DM present with microvascular complications at the time of diagnosis.

Obesity

Obesity is defined in terms of BMI and is calculated simply as the patient's weight in kilograms divided by the patient's height in meters squared: Weight (kg) ÷ Height (meters)^2

In general, the higher the BMI, the more insulin-resistant an individual is, with greater demands being placed on the already compromised pancreatic beta cell in the T2DM individual. In general, BMI correlates with percentage of body fat; however, in individuals with high muscle mass secondary to extensive physical training, the BMI may not accurately reflect body composition.

Metabolic Syndrome

Metabolic syndrome is frequently at the crossroads of T2DM and obesity. The diagnostic criteria for the metabolic syndrome per the National Cholesterol Education Program Adult Treatment Panel III are the presence of three of the following:[5]

1. Waist circumference >40 inches in men and >35 inches in women, taking into account ethnic adjustments
2. Blood pressure (BP) ≥130/85 mmHg
3. HDL-C <40 mg/dL in men and <50 mg/dL in women
4. Triglyceride levels ≥150 mg/dL
5. Fasting glucose ≥100 mg/dL

There has been some debate with regard to the value of diagnosing the metabolic syndrome on the grounds that it does not add to the overall risk of the individual elements compared to the total risk of the individual elements. The importance of the metabolic syndrome in clinical practice is that it should trigger the practitioner to look for other elements of the metabolic syndrome when even one element is present and especially alert the practitioner to diagnose T2DM earlier. For example, it is worthwhile to screen for T2DM in an individual with elevated triglycerides and low HDL-C.

Table 2.1 BMI Classifications	
BMI	**Classification**
<18.5	Underweight
18.5– 24.9	Normal
25–29.9	Overweight
30–39.9	Obesity
≥40	Morbid obesity

References

1. American Diabetes Association. Diagnosis and classification of diabetes mellitus. *Diabetes Care*. 2011;34(Suppl 1):S62-S69.

2. The International Expert Committee report on the role of the A1c assay in the diagnosis of diabetes. *Diabetes Care*. 2009;32(7):1327–1334.

3. American Association of Clinical Endocrinologists Board of Directors and American College of Endocrinology Board of Trustees. Statement on the use of hemoglobin A1c for the diagnosis of diabetes. *Endocrine Practice*. 2010;16(2):155–156.

4. Gale EAM. Declassifying diabetes. *Diabetalogia*. 2006;49(9):1989–1995.

5. Grundy SM, Brewer HB, Cleeman JI, et al. for the Conference Participants. Definition of metabolic syndrome. Report of the National Heart, Lung and Blood Institute/American Heart Association conference on scientific issues related to definition. *Circulation*. 2004;109:433–438.

Chapter 3

Pathophysiology

T2DM

T2DM is really a heterogeneous disorder involving variable degrees of insulin resistance and beta-cell and alpha-cell dysfunction.[1]

Insulin Resistance

Insulin resistance occurs at the level of the liver, the skeletal muscle, and the adipocyte.[2,3]

Liver

1. Uncontrolled hepatic glucose output in both the fasting and the fed state
2. Hypersecretion of triglyceride via very-low-density lipoprotein (VLDL)
3. Abnormal fat accumulation in the liver with resultant non-alcoholic steatohepatitis (NASH) and risk of cirrhosis.

Skeletal Muscle

1. Defective insulin-mediated glucose uptake by skeletal muscle
2. Defective non-oxidative glucose metabolism
3. Abnormal fat accumulation in skeletal muscle with resultant decreased ability to oxidize fatty acids
4. Questionable mitochondrial dysfunction[4]

Adipocyte

1. Increased lipolysis with enhanced release of free fatty acids (FFAs) and negative impact on insulin sensitivity elsewhere
2. Increased release of pro-inflammatory cytokines[2]
3. Decreased production of adiponectin, the only adipocytokine that has insulin sensitizing and anti-inflammatory properties. Indeed, low levels of adiponectin are predictive of future T2DM and coronary artery disease. In clinical trials, thiazolidinediones have been demonstrated to raise adiponectin levels.
4. Defective fat storage. Ectopic fat accumulation occurs in skeletal muscle and even more so in the liver as obesity progresses. Apoptosis of adipocytes results from the hypertrophy and hyperplasia of adipocytes in response to progressive obesity. The vascular system may not be able to adequately expand to maintain oxygenation and nutrition to the hypertrophic adipocyte, thus contributing to apoptosis. Release of pro-inflammatory cytokines and chemokines may attract circulating monocytes on the road to becoming macrophages. The adipocyte then becomes host to a self-perpetuating inflammatory cycle.

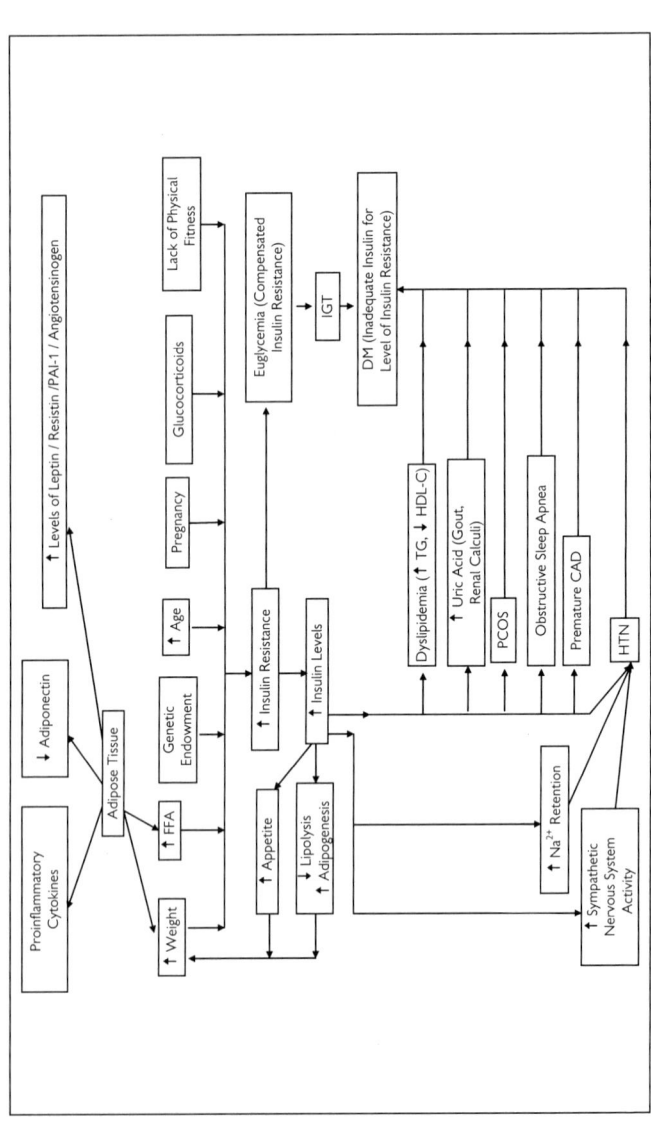

Figure 3.1 Insulin resistance

Beta-Cell Dysfunction

Beta-cell dysfunction has been noted for up to a decade prior to clinical presentation with T2DM. Defects include:

1. Loss of pulsatility of insulin secretion from the beta cell—a factor in hepatic insulin resistance
2. Loss of first-phase/early insulin release with resultant failure to rapidly shut off hepatic glucose production when ingesting carbohydrate
3. Progressive blunting of second phase of insulin secretion
4. Progressive beta-cell apoptosis with compromised beta-cell number and function. Beta-cell function is already reduced by as much as 80% at the time of diagnosis of T2DM, with loss thereafter at a rate of 4% to 6% per year, leading to progressive insulinopenia.[1]
5. Progressive beta-cell loss attributed to inflammation, glucotoxicity, and lipotoxicity[5]
6. Defective glucagon-like peptide-1 (GLP-1) signaling due largely to GLP-1 deficiency
7. Gastric inhibitory peptide (GIP) resistance
8. Amylin deficiency
9. The role of inflammation in beta-cell loss. Levels of both oxidized low-density lipoprotein (LDL) and interleukin-1ß, a pro-inflammatory cytokine that inhibits the function of beta cells and promotes their apoptosis, increase in response to hyperglycemia. In the beta cells of individuals with T2DM, the levels of interleukin-1-receptor antagonist, a natural antagonist of interleukin-1ß, are low, resulting in a pro-inflammatory state. Anakinra, a recombinant human interleukin-1-receptor antagonist, has been studied in 70 individuals with T2DM in a 13-week clinical trial, showing improved C-peptide levels, improved pro-insulin to insulin ratios, and better HbA1c values.[6] Markers of skeletal muscle insulin resistance did not improve during the trial, suggesting the HbA1c improvement was solely on the basis of improved beta-cell function. Recent studies suggest that oligomers of islet amyloid polypeptide trigger the generation of interleukin-1ß.[7] Furthermore, amyloid deposition is associated with progressive loss of beta-cell function.[8] Native GLP-1 has been shown to decrease islet apoptosis in cultured human islets.

Alpha-Cell Dysfunction

1. Dysregulation of glucagon secretion with failure to suppress glucagon with feeding, resulting in accelerated hepatic glucose production in both the fasting and the fed state
2. Hyperglucagonemia in part due to defective insulin signaling within the islet, deficiency of GLP-1, and amylin deficiency

Obesity

Obesity is a complex neuroendocrine and behavioral disorder related to a fundamental imbalance of energy intake versus energy expenditure. Obesity has both genetic and environmental components.

Genetic Factors

The genetic elements are complex and involve:

1. Leptin resistance with defective leptin transport across the blood–brain barrier
2. Probable central nervous system insulin resistance and defective signaling
3. Abnormalities in hypothalamic neuropeptide signaling
4. Ghrelin
5. Other gut peptides such as cholecystokinin (CCK)

Environmental Factors

Environmental factors involve both energy intake and energy expenditure.
Increased energy (food) intake factors include:

1. Stress-induced hyperphagia
2. Consumption of calorie-dense foods such as sweetened beverages that have limited/transient satiety
3. Food availability
   a. Food choices at work
   b. Food choices at home
   c. All-you-can-eat buffets
   d. Restaurant menu choices
   e. Restaurant portion sizes
   f. Snack packaging size
   g. Vending machines

4. Lack of personal culinary skills
   a. Skills not acquired at home/school
   b. Dependence on prepared foods from supermarkets
   c. Dependence on fast foods
   d. Failure to prepare meals from scratch at home

5. Lack of knowledge of the caloric values of foods, resulting in underestimation of caloric intake
6. Excessive alcohol intake with failure to compute calories ingested
7. Maintaining the higher caloric intake of pregnancy even in the postpartum period

Decreased energy expenditure factors include:

1. Global decrease in energy expenditure related to energy-sparing effects of:
   a. Automobiles versus walking/biking
   b. Elevators/escalators
   c. Drive-through services
   d. Office work versus farming/labor-intensive occupations

2. Failure to dedicate time for personal fitness and change negative views towards exercise. Personal fitness can include:
   a. Increased walking, reinforced by wearing a pedometer
   b. Use of home exercise equipment

c. Membership in local gymnasium/fitness center/recreation center programs
d. Engaging in various individual and team recreational sports
e. Use of video-enhanced recreational products
f. Dancing

Statistics on exercise are abysmal, with only 31% of adults reporting participation in regular leisure-time activity.[9]

References

1. Defronzo RA. From the triumvirate to the ominous octet: A new paradigm for the treatment of type 2 diabetes mellitus. *Diabetes.* 2009;58(4):773–795.

2. de Luca C, Olefsky JM. Inflammation and insulin resistance. *FEBS Lett.* 2008;582(1):97–105.

3. de Luca C, Olefsky JM. Stressed out about obesity and insulin resistance. *Nat Med.* 2006;12:41-42.

4. Højllund K, Mogensen M, Sahlin, K et al. Mitochondrial dysfunction in type 2 diabetes and obesity. *Endocrinol Metab Clin North Am.* 2008;37(3):713–731.

5. Karaca M, Magnan C, Karger C. Functional pancreatic beta-cell mass: Involvement in type 2 diabetes and therapeutic intervention. *Diabetes Metab.* 2009;35(2):77–84.

6. Larsen C, Faulenbach M, Vaag A et al. Interleukin-1-receptor antagonist in type 2 diabetes mellitus. *N Engl J Med.* 2007;356(15):1517–1526.

7. Masters SL, Dunne A, Subramanian SL, et al. Activation of the NLRP3 inflammasome by islet amyloid polypeptide provides a mechanism for enhanced IL-1ß in type 2 diabetes. *Nature Immunology.* 2010;11(10):897–904.

8. Clark A, Wells CA, Buley ID, et al. Islet amyloid, increased A-cells, reduced B-cells and exocrine fibrosis: Quantitative changes in the pancreas in type 2 diabetes. *Diabetes Res.* 1988;9(4):151–159.

9. U.S. Department of Health and Human Services, National Institutes of Health, National Institute of Diabetes and Digestive and Kidney Disease. *Statistics Related to Overweight and Obesity.* NIH Publication Number 04-4158. February 2010.

Chapter 4

Management of T2DM

Diabetes Education

An educated and motivated patient is the key to success in diabetes management. Patients need to understand the pathophysiology of T2DM and need to know that it is a progressive disorder requiring ongoing lifestyle changes as well as medication changes tailored to the progression of the disorder. Patients should also understand the coronary risk-equivalent nature of T2DM and the need for early intensive risk factor modification (IRFM). A clear understanding of all of these issues by the patient and reassurance from the clinician that clinical trials have shown reduction in both microvascular and macrovascular complications (as was seen in the landmark United Kingdom Prospective Diabetes Study [UKPDS][1]) will aid in optimal disease management, The "legacy effect" of antecedent poor glycemic control[2,3] needs to be addressed, as well as clinical inertia, whereby health care providers delay additional pharmacotherapy (especially insulin), resulting in persistently elevated HbA1c.

Diabetes education is critical to the success of a patient with T2DM. Certified Diabetes Educators (CDEs), health care professionals certified by the National Certification Board of Diabetes Educators, are critical to providing education and assisting in the translation of concepts into practice in patients' lives. CDEs may be hospital-based, as in American Diabetes Association (ADA)-certified diabetes programs, or physician office-based. To locate a CDE in your community, contact the American Association of Diabetes Educators.[4]

As data from new clinical trials emerge, ongoing reinforcement of the educational message is key, as is praise for incremental positive lifestyle changes. The many psychosocial obstacles to optimization of diabetes control need to be addressed. These include:

1. Cost of medications/co-pays for medications
2. Cost of blood glucose monitoring supplies
3. Cost of office visits/co-pays
4. Cost of nutrition counseling
5. Cost of diabetes self-management training
6. Concerns regarding absence from work for scheduled follow-up appointments, perhaps involving need to file paperwork for the Family Medical Leave Act (FMLA)
7. Stress and depression associated with dealing with a chronic illness

8. Other psychosocial obstacles to diabetes management, such as eating disorders
9. Cultural issues and communication problems related to language barriers and health beliefs

It is critical that all the obstacles to good care are identified and minimized.[5]

Monitoring Diabetes Control

Home blood glucose monitoring

Home blood glucose monitoring (HBGM) continues to become more rapid and reliable and less uncomfortable with the advancing technology of meters, strips, and lancing devices. The volume of blood required is frequently less than 1 μL and testing time is less than 5 seconds. Some glucose meters require no strip lot coding.

Frequency of HBGM may vary from once a day for a patient treated with lifestyle modification to 10 or more times per day for an insulinopenic patient who is on basal-bolus insulin therapy or insulin pump therapy. When a patient is monitoring only once a day, it is important to get both pre- and postprandial values to assess glycemic excursions. A sample test schedule might be: Sunday test pre-breakfast, Monday test 2 hours post-breakfast, Tuesday test pre-lunch, Wednesday test 2 hours post-lunch, Thursday test pre-dinner, Friday test 2 hours post-dinner, and Saturday test at bedtime.

Sources of error in HBGM include:

1. Failure to calibrate/code the meter
2. Failure to use control solution
3. Expired test strips
4. Test strips that have been damaged by cold, heat, light, or humidity
5. Inadequate lancing of the finger, which may lead the patient to apply excess pressure to express the blood, thus increasing the proportion of plasma component versus cellular component and increasing the glucose result (as glucose levels are higher in plasma than in whole blood)

Alternative-site testing, using a site other than the fingertips, can be successfully and safely used only when patients are fasting or have not eaten for 4 hours. Alternative-site testing should NEVER be used when glucose levels are rapidly changing, such as postprandially, or to confirm hypoglycemia, as the alternative-site test may underestimate the glucose result.

Patients need to review their blood glucose values in the context of food intake and activity to really understand the value of HBGM. This is a great learning opportunity for patients to understand the impact of both food intake and exercise on blood glucose levels.

Continuous Glucose Monitoring

Continuous glucose monitoring (CGM) continues to improve and currently is an adjunct to, not a replacement for, capillary fingerstick HBGM. The various CGM sensors currently on the U.S. market (Abbott Freestyle Navigator®,

DexCom Seven®Plus, and Medtronic Guardian REAL-Time®) all have to be calibrated with capillary fingerstick HBGM. CGM sensors are used generally only in insulin-treated patients. Clinical trials have generally focused on patients with T1DM. The Star-3 study showed encouraging results of sensor-augmented insulin pump therapy in individuals with T1DM, with greater HbA1c lowering (0.8% vs. 0.2%) without increased hypoglycemia.[6] CGM limitations include:

1. No reduction in the frequency of severe hypoglycemia
2. HbA1c reduction only in individuals with T1DM over the age of 25 years who wear the sensor 80% of the time[7]
3. Limited insurance coverage for most individuals for both the transmitter and sensors, thereby making it cost-prohibitive for many individuals
4. Many false alarms. Examples include (a) the hypoglycemia alarm going off when a confirmatory capillary fingerstick is in the euglycemic range, (b) loss of contact of the sensor with the transmitter, and (c) the need with some systems to set the transmitter hypoglycemia alarm parameter ≥85 mg/dL to reliably detect hypoglycemia.

CGM is FDA approved only for trend detection of hypoglycemia and hyperglycemia. The immediate CGM value CANNOT be used to adjust therapy, such as the dosing of insulin or treatment of hypoglycemia. It may be of value for patients with poor hypoglycemia awareness and those with a morbid fear of hypoglycemia. It is hoped that future generations of sensors will more reliably detect hypoglycemia and assist with improvement in HbA1c, and may do so at a lower cost and with better insurance coverage.

1, 5 Anhydroglucitol

Measurement of 1, 5 anhydroglucitol gives a measure of postprandial hyperglycemia. Postprandial hyperglycemia is especially relevant as patients are getting closer to goal HbA1c; in this range, the major contributor to the HbA1c result is the postprandial value rather than the pre-meal value. This test may complement the HbA1c and HBGM in selected patients. Postprandial metabolic disturbance may be a more important variable in microvascular and macrovascular complication risk than the fasting glucose level, given that most patients spend more of their 24-hour day in the postprandial rather than the fasting state.

Non-pharmacologic Treatment

Therapeutic Lifestyle Changes

Successful management of T2DM, obesity, and metabolic syndrome is critically dependent on therapeutic lifestyle changes (TLC). Diet and exercise in individuals with IGT resulted in a 58% risk reduction for the development of T2DM in the Diabetes Prevention Program Study (DPP); these lifestyle changes were superior in effect to metformin.[8] The Look-AHEAD (Action for Health in Diabetes) Trial in T2DM demonstrated a 0.7% HbA1c reduction with intensified diet and exercise programs in the first year.[9] This is comparable to the effect seen from adding one of several pharmacotherapeutic agents. Implementation me of TLC can be problematic, however, and it needs continuous reinforcement.

of TLC can be problematic, however, and it needs continuous reinforcement. The Look-AHEAD 4-year data illustrated this challenge, with the HbA1c reductions being less dramatic (−0.36% vs. 0.098%).[10] Additionally, the intensive lifestyle group exhibited better physical fitness, better systolic blood pressure, and higher HDL-C levels with better weight control. The hope is that those changes will result in decreased future cardiovascular events.

Medical Nutrition Therapy

Medical nutrition therapy (MNT) is the cornerstone of treatment for T2DM and should involve the use of CDEs, registered dietitians, and registered nurses, who can work with the patient on an ongoing basis. Nutrition information cannot be imparted in a one-shot deal. The fundamentals need to be addressed and then built upon to incorporate various subjects such as sodium and fiber intake. MNT in T2DM should focus on the concept of "meal plan" versus "diet." A "diet" is something one follows for a specified time period. A "meal plan" is a "plan for life."

The number of kCal in the meal plan depends upon the patient's ideal body weight (IBW), not the patient's current weight. Calculation of IBW can be performed by either the Hamwi formula or the Harris-Benedict equation. Calories for weight maintenance are also based on estimated usual energy expenditure. Most individuals with T2DM overestimate their energy expenditure, so unless the patient engages in heavy manual labor, there is little need to add calories to the calculation. In fact, for the majority of patients with T2DM, weight loss is needed, so calories should be subtracted to facilitate weight loss. There are 3,500 kCal in one pound of fat; therefore, to lose 1 lb/week a patient needs to achieve a caloric deficit of 500 kCal per day via decreased caloric intake and increased energy expenditure. Likewise, consuming an extra 100 kCal per day, which appears trivial to most patients, will result in an annual weight gain of 10 pounds.

A careful individualized intake assessment helps the health care team develop a meal plan that is appropriate for the individual. Individuals differ in their likes/dislikes, ethnic/cultural food preferences, meal timing, meal location, etc. A one-size-fits-all approach does not work in a chronic medical condition.[11] Tools for patients include books such as *The Calorie King® Calorie, Fat & Carbohydrate Counter*, which includes the weights/measures and nutrition content of various foods, as well as food scales and measuring cups for precise weighing and measuring. Food quantity is the major problem for most patients. Even if the food is healthy, if eaten in too large a portion, "good can lead to evil." When portion control is a problem, some patients find that commercial programs such as Weight Watchers®, Take Off Pounds Sensibly (TOPS)®, and Nutrisystem® provide them with the ease and consistency of healthy food in appropriate portion sizes. Others find Web-based nutrition programs helpful. What works for one patient does not necessarily work for another patient. Regardless of which particular plan is used, food logs can be helpful for both the health care provider and the patient to identify eating patterns, food choices, food quantities, etc. that positively or negatively affect the patient's health. Avoidance of fat-laden

is not applicable.

and calorie-laden foods such as chips and sweets is critical for weight loss, as is avoidance of the empty calories from alcohol.

Caveat: Most individuals underestimate their caloric intake and overestimate their energy expenditure.

Recidivism after any weight loss program is very problematic, with the most success being recorded in individuals who continue to exercise and maintain regular contact with the weight loss counseling team. Recent studies have suggested that a diet somewhat higher in protein and lower in glycemic index might be the best approach regarding maintenance of weight loss. Concern has been expressed that low-carbohydrate/high-protein diets may have adverse consequences in the long term in terms of death from cancer, cardiovascular disease, and indeed all-cause mortality.[12]

Exercise

Physical training has a profound impact on insulin sensitivity and metabolic control. Patients must understand that exercise capacity is a very important predictor of survival.[13,14] A program of progressive aerobic and resistance training will have even more profound effects than additional pharmacotherapy. The impact includes:

1. Reduction in body fat/body weight
2. Increase in muscle mass
3. Improved fasting and postprandial glycemic control
4. Improved HDL-C
5. Lower triglycerides
6. Improved insulin sensitivity
7. Improved cardiovascular fitness and aerobic capacity
8. Improved mood and overall well-being
9. Improved core strength and decreased propensity to fall
10. Reduced markers of inflammation[15]

A paradigm change needs to occur such that exercise becomes a priority in a given individual's life versus an elective issue. Patients must take time for exercise now, or be forced to take time off for illness in the future.

Strategies for incorporating exercise into an individual's daily routine include:

1. Walking more in the workplace—using stairs instead of the elevator
2. Use of a pedometer, with the daily goal of 10,000 steps per day. This goal is espoused by the ADA.
3. Home gym equipment
4. Recreation center/gymnasium membership
5. Personal trainer
6. Challenge programs within the workplace or social network

The key is ongoing motivation.

Caveat: In any patient who has coronary artery disease (CAD) or who is suspected of having CAD, cardiac evaluation is recommended before prescribing an exercise program.

Pathophysiologically Based Pharmacologic Interventions

Overview

Algorithms for the management of T2DM have been published by several professional organizations, including the ADA/European Association for the Study of Diabetes[16] and the American Association of Clinical Endocrinologists/ American College of Endocrinology,[17] with regular updates pending new clinical research.

Metformin should be the initial pharmacotherapy of choice, assuming there is no contraindication, and it should be initiated at the time of diagnosis in conjunction with diet and exercise. The durability of glycemic control varies significantly between the oral agents, with the least durability being seen with sulfonylureas and the greatest durability with the thiazoldinedione rosiglitazone.[18] Metformin appears intermediate in durability between sulfonylureas and rosiglitazone. Both oral and injectable incretin-based therapies hold promise of increased durability of glycemic control. This durability is probably related to better preservation of beta-cell function and decreased beta-cell apoptosis. Additionally, islet neogenesis has been documented in rodent models of diabetes with incretin-based therapies, but no human data exist.

If in 3 months the patient is not at HbA1c goal, then an additional agent should be prescribed. The majority of individuals will eventually require combination pharmacotherapy to achieve the goal HbA1c level. Using combination pharmacotherapy at submaximal doses addressing the different pathophysiological defects while attempting to minimize side effects yields the best response. Agent selection involves the consideration of:

1. Degree of HbA1c lowering needed
2. Residual beta-cell function
3. Comorbidities: gastrointestinal disorders, congestive heart failure (CHF), renal insufficiency, etc.
4. Risk of hypoglycemia
5. Risk of weight gain
6. Cost of medication/co-pays

The ideal treatment combination should achieve the goal HbA1c while minimizing weight gain and hypoglycemia. In this regard, many patients do well on a combination of metformin, thiazolidinedione, and incretin-based therapy. Sulfonylurea-based therapies have generally fallen out of favor for early use due to issues of lack of durability of glycemic control, weight gain, and hypoglycemia.

Oral Agents

A wide variety of oral agents are available. These agents address different physiologic defects and are complementary. Initial monotherapy with most oral agents in drug-naïve patients lowers the HbA1c 0.8% to 2.0%, and occasionally more. Combination therapy with agents having complementary modes of action will lower HbA1c an additional 0.5% to 2.0%.

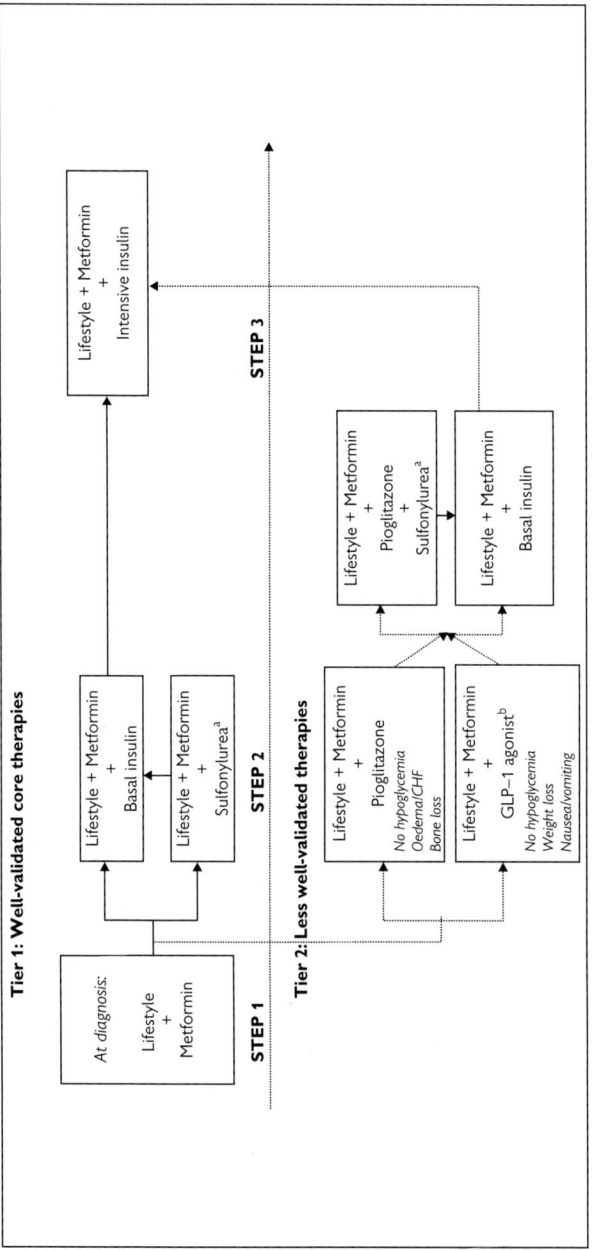

Figure 4.1 Algorithm for the metabolic management of type 2 diabetes. (Reprinted with permission from Nathan DM, Buse JB, Davidson MB, et al. Medical management of hyperglycemia in type 2 diabetes: a consensus algorithm for the initiation and adjustment of therapy. *Diabetes Care.* 2009;32(1):193–203.)

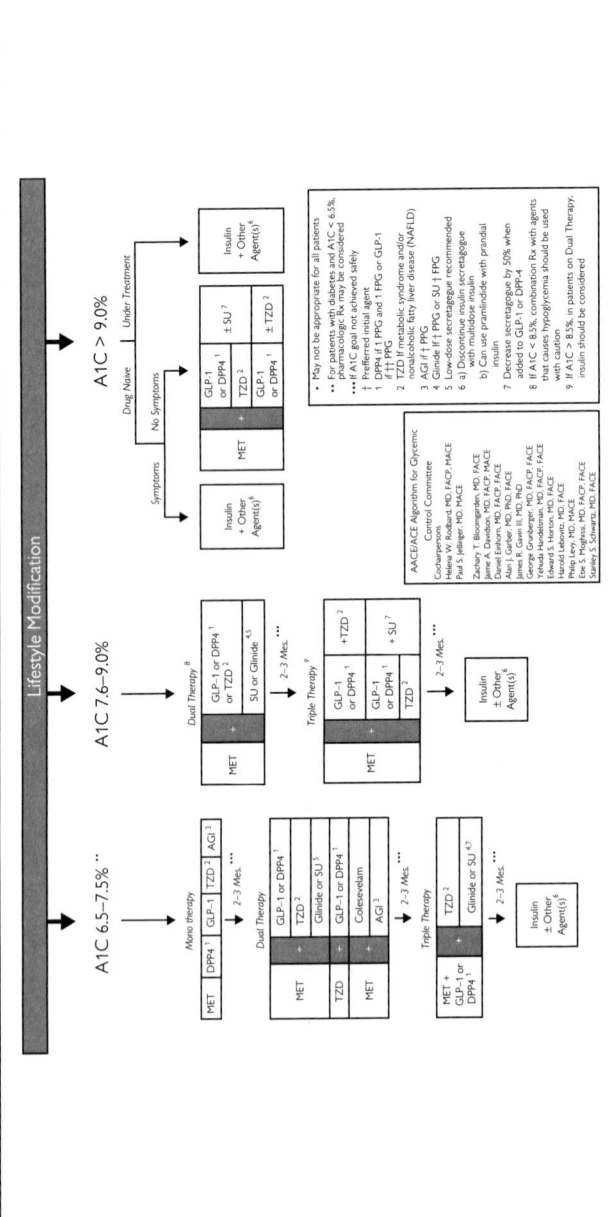

Figure 4.2 Diabetes algorithm for glycemic control. (Reprinted with permission from Rodbard HW, Jellinger PS, Davidson JA, et al. Statement by an American Association of Clinical Endocrinologists/American College of Endocrinology Consensus Panel on Type 2 Diabetes Mellitus. *Endocr Pract.* 2009;15(6): 541–559.)

Comparable glucose-lowering efficacy exists between rosiglitazone and pioglitazone, but pioglitazone appears to have better HDL-C–raising and triglyceride-lowering potential. Both agents appear to alter LDL-C from small, dense, readily oxidized particles to larger, more buoyant, and less atherogenic particles.

Controversy exists with regard to whether rosiglitazone causes increased coronary ischemic risk.[19] The hypothesis-generating meta-analysis of short-term clinical trials with unknown baseline risk suggests increased ischemic risk when the comparator agent was placebo (rather than other agents). Prescription database studies have yielded conflicting results when rosiglitazone is compared to pioglitazone, with the most recent database analysis suggesting comparable cardiovascular events between rosiglitazone and pioglitazone. The randomized clinical trials, on the other hand, which include RECORD (Rosiglitazone Evaluated for Cardiovascular Outcomes),[20] VADT (Glucose Control and Vascular Complications in Veterans with Type 2 Diabetes),[21] ACCORD (Action to Control Cardiovascular Risk in Diabetes),[22] and BARI 2D (Bypass Angioplasty Revascularization in 2 Diabetes),[23] failed to show any increased ischemic risk with rosiglitazone compared to other agents. Indeed, the BARI 2D *post-hoc* analysis showed a 28% relative risk reduction for cardiovascular events and mortality in favor of rosiglitazone.

The FDA has recently added restrictions to the use of rosiglitazone. Existing patients may continue to use the drug, assuming good clinical response. Patients should not be started on rosiglitazone unless there is no therapeutic alternative. A Risk Evaluation and Mitigation Strategy (REMS) program has been developed.

In June, 2011, the FDA issued a warning based on new data in regard to cumulative exposure with pioglitazone and the risk of bladder cancer. It is therefore prudent to discontinue pioglitazone in patients with active bladder cancer and perhaps also in patients with a prior history of bladder cancer.

Bromocriptine mesylate, a dopamine receptor agonist, was approved by the FDA in May 2009 as an adjunct to diet and exercise in adults with T2DM. The initial dose is 0.8 mg daily with food 2 hours after waking, with weekly dose titration as tolerated to the maximum dose of 4.8 mg daily (6 tablets). The CYP3A4 pathway is the major metabolic pathway, so caution is need when used concurrently with inducers, inhibitors, or substrates of the CYP3A4 pathway such as erythromycin, azole antimycotics, and protease inhibitors. HbA1c reductions have been modest (≤0.5%) in the clinical trials versus placebo. Common side effects include dizziness, fatigue, nausea, vomiting, and headaches; these resulted in relatively high discontinuation rates in the clinical trials. Cardiovascular safety has been documented in a 52-week clinical trial.[24] Significant weight loss has not been documented in human trials.

Injectable Incretin-Based Therapies

Exenatide

Exenatide has been on the market for 5 years. It has approximately 50% homology with native GLP-1 and is resistant to degradation by the DPP-IV enzyme. Therapy is initiated with 5 mcg SC b.i.d. using a pen injection device; the dose is escalated after 4 weeks to the optimal dose of 10 mcg bid, assuming no adverse effects from the lower dose. The most common side effects, nausea

Table 4.1 Oral Agents

	Metformin	Rosiglitazone	Pioglitazone	Sitagliptin	Saxagliptin	Linagliptin
Mode of action (MOA)	Primary MOA is ↓ hepatic glucose	↑ skeletal muscle glucose uptake ↓ free fatty acids	↑ skeletal muscle glucose uptake ↓ free fatty acids	Inhibition of dipeptidyl peptidase IV (DPP-IV), enzyme involved in degradation of GLP-1, resulting in a return to physiologic GLP-1 levels	Inhibition of dipeptidyl peptidase IV (DPP-IV), enzyme involved in degradation of GLP-1, resulting in a return to physiologic GLP-1 levels	Inhibition of dipeptidyl peptidase IV (DPP-IV), enzyme involved in degradation of GLP-1, resulting in a return to physiologic GLP-1 levels
Glucose effects	Mainly fasting	Fasting and postprandial	Fasting and postprandial	Mainly postprandial with lesser fasting effect	Mainly postprandial with lesser fasting effect	Mainly postprandial with lesser fasting effect
Hypoglycemia as monotherapy	No	No	No	No	No	No
Weight gain	No	Yes	Yes	No	No	No
Insulin levels	↓	↓	↓	↑ postprandially via glucose-dependent insulin secretion	↑ postprandially via glucose-dependent insulin secretion	↑ postprandially via glucose-dependent insulin secretion
Side effects	Self-limiting GI: diarrhea, nausea, anorexia minimized with extended-release (ER) preparations; vitamin B12 malabsorption	Weight gain, edema, congestive heart failure	Weight gain, edema, congestive heart failure	Upper respiratory infection, headache	Upper respiratory infection, urinary tract infection, headache	Upper respiratory infection
Lipid effects	↓ triglycerides	↑HDL-C ↓triglycerides ↓small dense LDL ↑LDL-C concentration	↑HDL-C ↓triglycerides ↓small dense LDL ↓LDL-C concentration	Neutral	Neutral	Neutral

Starting dose for a 70-kg man	500 mg bid of immediate-release (IR) 2 × 500 mg ER qpm	4 mg daily as single or divided dose	15 mg qd	Pending creatinine clearance (CrCl) <30 mL/min: 25 mg qd; 30–49 mL/min: 50 mg qd; ≥50 mL/min: 100 mg qd	2.5 mg qd if CrCl ≤50 mL/min or if co-administration with strong inhibitor of CYP3A4/5 such as clarithromycin; 5 mg qd if CrCl >50 mL/min	5 mg qd No dose reduction for renal or hepatic impairment
Maximum dose	850 mg IR tid 4 × 500 mg ER qpm	8 mg daily as a single or divided dose	45 mg qd	Pending CrCl <30 mL/min: 25 mg qd; 30–49 mL/min: 50 mg qd; ≥50 mL/min: 100 mg qd	2.5 mg qd if CrCl ≤50 mL/min or if co-administration with strong inhibitor of CYP3A4/5 such as clarithromycin; 5 mg qd if CrCl >50 mL/min	5 mg qd No dose reduction for renal or hepatic impairment
Contra-indications	T1DM, renal dysfunction, hepatic dysfunction, history of EtOH abuse, chronic conditions associated with hypoxia such as asthma, COPD, CHF, acute conditions associated with potential for hypoxia (surgery, acute MI, CHF), situations associated with potential renal dysfunction (IV contrast)	T1DM Edema/CHF	T1DM Edema/CHF	T1DM	T1DM	T1DM

(continued)

Table 4.1 (Cont.)

	Sulfonylureas	Repaglinide	Nateglinide	Acarbose	Miglitol	Colesevelam
Mode of action (MOA)	↑ insulin secretion	↑ insulin secretion	↑ insulin secretion	α-glucosidase inhibition resulting in ↓ carbohydrate digestion and absorption from GI tract	α-glucosidase inhibition resulting in ↓ carbohydrate digestion and absorption from GI tract	Unknown; may enhance insulin sensitivity
Glucose effects	Fasting and postprandial	Fasting and postprandial	Postprandial	Postprandial	Postprandial	Fasting in combination with metformin or sulfonylurea; A1c lowering in combination with metformin, sulfonylurea. or insulin
Hypoglycemia as monotherapy	Yes	Yes; less than that seen with sulfonylureas	Yes; less than that seen with repaglinide	No	No	No monotherapy indication
Weight gain	Yes	No	No	No	No	No
Insulin levels	↑	↑	↑	↓	↓	Neutral
Side effects	Potential allergic reaction if sulfa allergy; potential drug interactions with first-generation agents (chlorpropamide → SIADH)	None; equal to placebo	None; equal to placebo	GI (flatulence, abdominal distention, diarrhea)	GI (flatulence, abdominal distention, diarrhea)	Constipation

Lipid effects	↑ or ↓	Neutral	Neutral	↓	↓	↓ LDL-C ↑ triglycerides in insulin-treated patients
Starting dose for a 70-kg man	Varies with each agent Glyburide 2.5 mg qd Glipizide ER 5 mg qd Micronized glyburide 3 mg qd Glimepiride 2 mg qd	0.5 mg prior to meals	120 mg tid	25 mg tid with the first bite of each meal	25 mg tid with the first bite of each meal	3 g at lunch and dinner or 6 g with dinner
Maximum dose	Varies with each agent Glyburide 10 mg bid Glipizide ER 20 mg qd Micronized glyburide 6 mg bid Glimepiride 8 mg qd	16 mg daily in divided doses prior to meals	120 mg tid	100 mg tid	100 mg tid	3 g at lunch and dinner or 6 g with dinner
Contraindications	T1DM	T1DM; co-administration of gemfibrozil due to an increased repaglinide exposure	T1DM; caution in moderate or severe hepatic impairment due to no studies being available	T1DM, inflammatory bowel disease, bowel obstruction, cirrhosis, chronic conditions with maldigestion or malabsorption	T1DM, inflammatory bowel disease, bowel obstruction, cirrhosis, chronic conditions with maldigestion or malabsorption	Triglycerides > 500 mg/dl

and bloating, can be minimized by initially taking the medication 10 to 15 minutes before a meal. If nausea and bloating still occur, then it should be taken closer to the meal. Later, the dosing interval can be extended out as far as 60 minutes for optimization of early satiety and weight loss, assuming no excess nausea. Exenatide has the following attributes:

1. Restoration of first-phase (early) insulin secretion
2. Glucose-dependent augmentation of the second phase of insulin secretion
3. Suppression of hyperglucagonemia
4. Delayed gastric emptying
5. Promotion of central satiety
6. Weight loss is seen in approximately 75% of patients; this helps motivate ongoing patient adherence.

In addition to the benefits to glucose control and weight, exenatide has been shown to have a positive impact on blood pressure and triglycerides.

Patients who also take medications that are dependent upon threshold concentrations (e.g., antibiotics and oral contraceptives) should take those medications at least 1 hour prior to the administration of exenatide. Patients who take oral medications that must be taken with food should take them at meals/snacks when exenatide is not administered.

Adverse effects other than nausea, dyspepsia, occasional emesis, and diarrhea are uncommon. Post-marketing associations have been made with pancreatitis, so exenatide should be avoided in any patient with a history of pancreatitis and discontinued if pancreatitis is suspected. The incidence of pancreatitis in T2DM patients is felt to be approximately three times that of the general population via multiple mechanisms, including hypertriglyceridemia, increased cholelithiasis, and perhaps alcohol excess. Cholelithiasis *per se* should not be a contraindication to incretin-based therapies, as the annual risk of pancreatitis is quite low (0.05–2.0%).[25] Reports of renal failure in association with exenatide use have been made, which stresses the need to avoid exenatide in any patient with a creatinine clearance of <30 mL/min. It is important to recognize that these are associations and not causality; patients need reassurance in this regard.

Glycemic efficacy data suggest that the addition of exenatide to pre-existing oral agent therapy may be comparable to adding basal insulin without the weight gain frequently associated with basal insulin. Discontinuation of exenatide after 52 weeks of therapy results in a rapid loss (within 4 weeks) of the improvement in beta-cell function, so this therapy needs to be ongoing.

A once-weekly preparation has been submitted to the FDA for review. The Duration-1 Study compared the once-weekly exenatide preparation with the b.i.d. preparation and found that the once-weekly preparation resulted in better FPG and HbA1c values, with comparable weight loss and no increase in hypoglycemia.[26] The Duration-3 Study compared the once-weekly 2-mg exenatide preparation with insulin glargine and found a lower HbA1c, less hypoglycemia, better 1,5 anyhydroglucitol, and weight loss with exenatide versus superior FPG levels and progressive weight gain with insulin glargine.[27]

Liraglutide

Liraglutide is an analog of native GLP-1, with 97% homology to human GLP-1. It has a fatty acid side chain to enhance albumin binding, which gives liraglutide a half-life of approximately 13 hours and allows for once-daily dosing. Unlike exenatide, liraglutide does not have to be dosed in relationship to meals. The dominant side effect is nausea, similar to exenatide. The nausea abates over time, and with the dose titration via the pen device of 0.6 mg daily for the first week, 1.2 mg daily for the second week, and 1.8 mg daily thereafter if needed, patients rarely discontinue therapy. In the LEAD-3 monotherapy trial, the rate of nausea was comparable to glimepiride after 12 weeks.[28] The LEAD-5 study showed comparable HbA1c reduction to basal insulin when added to dual oral-agent therapy without attendant weight gain and with less risk of hypoglycemia.[29]

In a head-to-head trial of liraglutide versus exenatide (LEAD-6), liraglutide was associated with greater decrements in fasting blood glucose and superior HbA1c reduction (1.12% vs. 0.79%) with comparable weight loss. The post-breakfast and post-dinner blood glucose values were superior with exenatide b.i.d.[30]

Patients need to be aware of the association of C-cell hyperplasia with medullary thyroid cancer in rats and mice, though there are no cases recorded in monkeys or humans. A recent clinical review of calcitonin levels that were monitored for over 2 years in over 5,000 subjects with T2DM or non-diabetic obese subjects did not show any adverse effect of liraglutide on calcitonin levels. This is certainly reassuring and suggests that rodent data are not applicable to humans.[31] Liraglutide is contraindicated in patients with (1) a personal or family history of medullary thyroid cancer or (2) multiple endocrine neoplasia 2 (MEN 2) syndrome. Routine screening of calcitonin levels and screening thyroid ultrasound examinations are not indicated. Should a palpable thyroid nodule be found, then referral to an endocrinologist for ultrasound-guided fine-needle aspiration of the nodule would be appropriate. Because liraglutide delays gastric emptying, there is the potential for it to affect the absorption of concomitantly administered oral medications. However, in pharmacologic trials studying the effects of liraglutide on the absorption of certain oral medications, there was no significant effect.

Pramlintide

Pramlintide is a synthetic analog of the neuroendocrine hormone amylin, which is co-secreted with insulin by the beta cells in response to food intake. Pramlintide regulates glucose appearance in the bloodstream via regulation of gastric emptying and suppresses postprandial glucagon secretion. Pramlintide has no effect on insulin secretion. Pramlintide is dosed in either vials or via a pen device. Initial dosing is 60 mcg SC immediately prior to each major meal consisting of ≥30 g carbohydrate or ≥250 kCal. If no significant nausea has occurred for 3 to 7 days, the dose can be increased to 120 mcg SC. It is imperative to reduce the dose of certain insulins (rapid-acting analog [RAA], human regular insulin, or premixed insulin) by 50% when starting pramlintide to avoid hypoglycemia. There is a risk of insulin-induced severe hypoglycemia that can occur within 3 hours of the injection. Pramlintide is contraindicated in patients with an estimated creatinine clearance of <30 mL/min. Concomitant oral medications requiring rapid onset should be taken 1 hour before or 2 hours after pramlintide.

Insulin Therapy

Given the natural history of progressive loss of beta-cell function over time, insulin therapy will be inevitable for the majority of T2DM patients after 12 to 15 years with the disease.

Indications for Insulin Therapy
1. Failure to achieve glycemic goals with oral therapy with or without injected incretin-based therapies
2. Acute metabolic decompensation with polydipsia, polyuria, and/or weight loss
3. Acute illness with hyperglycemia

Goals of Insulin Therapy
1. Re-establish glycemic control and get patients to goal HbA1c
2. Minimize risk of hypoglycemia
3. Minimize weight gain

Insulin Regimen Options
1. Add basal insulin (detemir or glargine).
2. Add premixed insulin.
3. Add pre-meal (RAA) insulin (aspart/glulisine/lispro).
4. Add basal and pre-meal insulin.
5. Continuous subcutaneous insulin infusion (CSII)—insulin pump therapy.

Data from the recent 4T study suggests superiority of a basal insulin-based regimen in terms of HbA1c, weight gain, and hypoglycemia. Curiously, fewer cardiovascular events were noted in the basal insulin group.[32]

Insulin may be initiated at a dose of either (1) 10 units of basal insulin or (2) 0.2 units/kg of basal insulin at h.s. Additionally, the patient is then given a self-titration algorithm such as:
1. Every other night, increase insulin in 2-unit increments until fasting blood glucose is <110 mg/dL; or
2. Every three nights, increase insulin in 3-unit increments until fasting blood glucose is <110 mg/dL.

A follow-up visit after 1 week of insulin initiation is prudent to assess the clinical response. If there is has been little or no impact on the fasting hyperglycemia, then dose escalation to 0.3 units/kg should be considered. Many individuals need a final dose closer to 0.4 units/kg.

Clinical trials suggest that the addition of basal insulin will result in approximately 60% of patients reaching an HbA1c goal of <7.0%.[33,34] The remaining patients will have postprandial hyperglycemia as the problem. Generally consideration should be given to adding prandial RAA insulin when the 2-hour postprandial blood glucose levels are consistently ≥160 mg/dL. The more carbohydrate consumed at a meal, the higher the RAA dose needed to prevent hyperglycemia. Frequently, the evening meal is the largest carbohydrate-containing meal of the day and is therefore the first meal requiring the addition of RAA insulin. Later, as beta-cell function deteriorates, patients will need prandial insulin to cover other meals, such that the final outcome will be full multiple daily insulin injections (MDI). RAA insulin to carbohydrate ratios vary significantly between individuals. Leaner T2DM patients may achieve good postprandial glycemic control with an RAA insulin to carbohydrate ratio of 1 unit RAA for every 20 grams of carbohydrate at meals/snacks, while more insulin-resistant T2DM patients may need 1 unit RAA for every 3 grams of carbohydrate at meals/snacks. Individualization is the key!

An alternative plan in patients with fixed meal times and fixed carbohydrate intake would be to use a premixed insulin product. The downside of premixed insulin preparations is the tendency for more hypoglycemia and weight gain when the insulin is titrated aggressively to achieve tight glycemic goals.[35] In situations in which tight glycemic goals may not be an issue, such as advanced age and limited life expectancy (i.e., a nursing home patient), premixed insulin might be a valid option.

An occasional patient might have good FPGs on oral agents, yet have postprandial hyperglycemia. These patients need only prandial insulin and can use RAA matched to planned carbohydrate intake at meals and snacks.

Insulin Pump Therapy

CSII therapy may be an option for select insulinopenic T2DM patients who are failing basal-bolus therapy with MDI. Patients must realize that an insulin pump is NOT a panacea for diabetes and requires significant time and effort to derive optimal benefit. This effort is no less, and in fact more, than that required for MDI. Several health insurance carriers follow the Medicare criteria for insulin pump coverage for T2DM patients, to include:

1. A C-peptide value that is ≤110% of the lower limit of the normal laboratory measurement. The C-peptide value must be in the context of a simultaneous FPG of ≤225 mg/dL.
2. Positive islet cell cytoplasmic antibodies

The complexities of insulin pump therapy require good cognitive skills and documented commitment to optimal self-care. Assuming those criteria are met, insulinopenic T2DM patients can have optimization of glycemic control along with the freedom and flexibility that insulin pump therapy affords.

Insulin Pen Devices

Insulin pen devices can greatly facilitate adherence to MDI versus utilization of vial and syringe. Additionally, pen devices may be a lot less intimidating than a vial and syringe for patients initiating insulin therapy. Modern pen devices require less injection pressure/force than the earlier models, and with needle gauges as fine as 32G, the discomfort is truly negligible. To ensure correct and reliable dosing, patients need to be attentive to proper technique:

1. Adequate initial priming of a new pen
2. Adequate subsequent priming of pen with at least 2 units prior to each injection
3. Accurate dialing of insulin dose

4. Stretching of skin for a clean puncture instead of pinching. Pinching can cause efflux of insulin after needle removal.
5. Counting to 10 prior to removing the needle to minimize any back-seepage/dribbling and subsequent loss of insulin
6. Changing needle with each use and NOT storing the needle attached to the pen

Limitations of pen devices include the volume of insulin per pen (300 units for all pen devices) and the number of units per injection that can be administered (varies per manufacturer). Individuals taking high doses of insulin typically utilize vial/syringe. Unfortunately, the per-unit cost of insulin in a pen device is higher than that in a vial, such that some health insurance carriers will either charge patients a higher-tier co-pay for pen devices or not reimburse for pen devices altogether, despite the opportunity to enhance patient acceptability and adherence to insulin therapy. Since inadequate insulinization leads to inadequate glycemic control with attendant consequences, the optimization of patient adherence should be the goal of therapy. The pen device being used can be stored at temperature <85°F; additional pen devices should be kept refrigerated. Exposure to temperature extremes (heat or cold) can result in denaturation of the insulin, loss of efficacy, and hyperglycemia.

References

1. UK Prospective Diabetes Study (UKPDS) Group. Intensive blood-glucose control with sulphonylureas or insulin compared with conventional treatment and risk of complications in patients with type 2 diabetes (UKPDS 33). *Lancet.* 1998;352(9131):837–853.
2. Holman RR, Paul SK, Bethal MA, et al. 10-year follow-up of intensive glucose control in type 2 diabetes. *N Engl J Med.* 2008;359(15):1577–1589.
3. Chalmers J, Cooper ME. UKPDS and the legacy effect. *N Engl J Med.* 2008;359(15):1618–1620.
4. American Association of Diabetes Educators. Find a diabetes educator. http://diabeteseducator.org/find.
5. Sheehan JP. Bad medicine: There is a lot wrong with diabetes care in the United States. *Cult Med Pyschiatry.* 2010;34:2–12.
6. Bergenstal RM, Tamborlane WV, Ahman A, et al. Effectiveness of sensor-augmented insulin pump therapy in type 1 diabetes. *N Engl J Med.* 2010;363(4):311–320.
7. The Juvenile Diabetes Research Foundation Continuous Glucose Monitoring Study Group. Continuous glucose monitoring and intensive treatment of type 1 diabetes. *N Engl J Med.* 2008;359(14):1464–1476.
8. Diabetes Prevention Program Research Group. Reduction in the incidence of type 2 diabetes with lifestyle intervention or metformin. *N Engl J Med.* 2002;346(6):393–403.
9. The Look AHEAD Research Group. Reduction in weight and cardiovascular disease risk factors in individuals with type 2 diabetes: The one-year results of the Look AHEAD trial. *Diabetes Care.* 2007;30(6):1374–1383.

10. The Look AHEAD Research Group. Long-term effects of a lifestyle intervention on weight and cardiovascular risk factors in individuals with type 2 diabetes mellitus. Four-year results of the Look AHEAD trial. *Arch Intern Med.* 2010;170(17):1566–1575.

11. Sacks FM, Bray GA, Carey VJ, et al. Comparison of weight-loss diets with different compositions of fat, protein, and carbohydrates. *N Engl J Med.* 2009;360(9):859–873.

12. Fung TT, van Dam RM, Hankinson SE, et al. Low-carbohydrate diets and all-cause and cause-specific mortality. Two cohort studies. *Ann Intern Med.* 2010;153(5):289–298.

13. Myers J, Prakash M, Froelicher V, et al. Exercise capacity and mortality among men referred for exercise testing. *N Engl J Med.* 2002;346(11):763–801.

14. Gulati M, Pandey DK, Arnsdorf MF, et al. Exercise capacity and the risk of death in women: The St. James Women Take Heart project. *Circulation.* 2003;108(13):1554–1559.

15. Milani RV, Lavie CJ, Mehra MR. Reduction in C-reactive protein through cardiac rehabilitation and exercise training. *J Am Coll Cardiol.* 2004;43(6):1056–1061.

16. Nathan DM, Buse JB, Davidson MB, et al. for the American Diabetes Association, European Association for the Study of Diabetes. Medical management of hyperglycemia in type 2 diabetes: A consensus algorithm for the initiation and adjustment of therapy. A consensus statement of the American Diabetes Association and the European Association for the Study of Diabetes. *Diabetes Care.* 2009;32(1):193–203.

17. Rodbard HW, Jellinger PS, Davidson JA. Statement by American Association of Clinical Endocrinologists/American College of Endocrinology consensus panel on type 2 diabetes mellitus: An algorithm for glycemic control. *Endocr Pract.* 2009;15(6):540–557.

18. Kahn SE, Haffner SM, Heise MA for the ADOPT Study Group. Glycemic durability of rosiglitazone, metformin, or glyburide monotherapy. *N Engl J Med.* 2006;355(23):2427–2443.

19. Rosen CJ. Revisiting the rosiglitazone story—Lessons learned. *N Engl J Med.* 2010;363(9):803–806.

20. Home PD, Pocock SJ, Beck-Nielsen H, et al. for the RECORD Study Group. Rosiglitazone Evaluated for Cardiovascular Outcomes—An interim analysis. *N Engl J Med.* 2007;357(1):28–38.

21. Duckworth W, Abraira C, Moritz T, et al. Glucose control and vascular complication in veterans with type 2 diabetes. *N Engl J Med.* 2009;360(2):129–139.

22. The Action to Control Cardiovascular Risk in Diabetes Study Group. Effect of intensive glucose lowering in type 2 diabetes. *N Engl J Med.* 2008;358(24):2545–2559.

23. Bach RG, Lombardero M, Brooks MM, et al. Rosiglitazone and outcomes for patients with diabetes and coronary artery disease in the BARI 2D Trial. Late-breaking clinical study presented at the 70th Scientific Sessions of the American Diabetes Association, 2010, Orlando, Florida.

24. Gaziano JM, Cincotta AH, O'Connor CM, et al. Randomized clinical trial of quick-release bromocriptine among patients with type 2 diabetes on overall safety and cardiovascular outcomes. *Diabetes Care.* 2010;33(7):1503–1508.

25. Venneman NG, Buskens E, Besselink MGH, et al. Small gallstones are associated with increased risk of acute pancreatitis: Potential benefits of prophylactic cholecystectomy? *Am J Gastroenterol.* 2005;100(11):2540–2550.

26. Drucker DJ, Buse JB, Taylor K, et al. Exenatide once weekly versus twice daily for the treatment of type 2 diabetes: A randomized, open-label, non-inferiority study. *Lancet.* 2008;372(9645):1240–1250.

27. Diamant M, Van Gaal L, Strank S, et al. Once-weekly exenatide compared with insulin glargine titrated to target in patients with type 2 diabetes (Duration-3): An open-label randomized trial. *Lancet.* 2010;375(9733):2234–2243.

28. Garber A, Henry R, Ratner R, et al. Liraglutide versus glimepiride monotherapy for type 2 diabets (LEAD-3 Mono): A randomized, 52-week, phase III, double-blind parallel treatment trial. *Lancet.* 2009;373(9662):473–481.

29. Rusell-Jones D, Vaag A, Schmitz O, et al. Liraglutide vs. insulin glargine and placebo in combination with metformin and sulfonylurea therapy in type 2 diabetes mellitus (LEAD-5 met+su): A randomized controlled trial. *Diabetalogia.* 2009;52(10):2046–2055.

30. Buse JB, Rosenstock J, Sesti G, et al. Liraglutide once a day vs. exenatide twice a day for type 2 diabetes: A 26-week randomized, parallel-group, multinational, open-label trial (LEAD-6). *Lancet.* 2009;374(9683):39–47.

31. Hegedüs L, Moses AC, Zdravkovic M, et al. GLP-1 and calcitonin concentration in humans: Lack of evidence of calcitonin release from sequential screening in over 5000 subjects with type 2 diabetes or nondiabetic obese subjects treated with the human GLP-1 analog, liraglutide. *J Clin Endocrin Metab.* 2011;96(3):853–860.

32. Holman RR, Farmer AJ, Davies MJ, et al. Three-year efficacy of complex insulin regimens in type 2 diabetes. *N Engl J Med.* 2009;361(18):1736–1747.

33. Riddle, MC, Rosenstock, J, Gerich J. The treat-to-target trial: Randomized addition of glargine or human NPH insulin to oral therapy of type 2 diabetic patients. *Diabetes Care.* 2003;26(11):3080–3086.

34. Philis-Tsimikas A, Charpentier G, Clausen P, et al. Comparison of once-daily insulin detemir with NPH insulin added to a regimen of oral antidiabetic drugs in poorly controlled type 2 diabetes. *Clin Ther.* 2006;28(10):1569–1581.

35. Raskin P, Allen E, Hollander P, et al. Initiating insulin therapy in type 2 diabetes: A comparison of biphasic and basal insulin analogs. *Diabetes Care.* 2005;28(2):260–265.

Chapter 5

Management of Obesity: Implications for T2DM

Pharmacotherapy

The central role of obesity in insulin resistance, hypertension, and dyslipidemia makes it an attractive target for pharmacotherapy. The ideal agent would both reduce weight and prevent the development of T2DM, control associated cardiovascular risk factors, and significantly improve glycemic control without significant adverse effects.

The use of orlistat in this regard has only had modest success and has been limited by gastrointestinal side effects and significant cost.[1]

The serotonin reuptake inhibitors fenfluramine and dexfenfluramine, the latter of which also promotes presynaptic serotonin release, held considerable promise. The weight loss with these agents was modest and required continuous use to maintain weight loss. Unfortunately, these agents caused significant valvulopathy similar to that seen with other serotonergic agents, such as pergolide and cabergoline, and to that seen in patients with the carcinoid syndrome. Pulmonary hypertension was also seen and was frequently fatal. Further studies identified that activation of the $5HT_{2B}$ receptor in cardiac valvular interstitial cells was probably the cause. Fenfluramine and dexfenfluramine were removed from the U.S. market by the FDA in 1997.

More selective serotonin receptor agonists such as lorcaserin, a $5HT_{2C}$ agonist, hold promise for the future. A recent clinical trial of this agent versus placebo in obese non-diabetic individuals revealed significant weight loss and reductions in blood pressure, LDL-C, triglycerides, fasting glucose, fasting insulin, HbA1c, and high-sensitivity C-reactive protein without any evidence of valvulopathy.[2] The FDA advisory committee recently voted against approval and will require more extensive safety and efficacy data.

Sibutramine is a combined serotonin and norepinephrine reuptake inhibitor approved for the management of obesity. This agent causes modest weight loss and must be used continuously to maintain weight loss. Blood pressure elevation is a significant side effect that needs careful monitoring. Unfortunately, the large long-term cardiovascular outcome clinical trial in patients with T2DM and coronary artery disease proved disappointing, with increased stroke and myocardial infarction in sibutramine-treated patients.[3] Sibutramine has since been withdrawn from the market.

A combination product, Contrave, containing bupropion and naltrexone, received an approval vote from the FDA advisory panel in December 2010. Concern was expressed regarding possible adverse effects on blood pressure and potential for seizures. The FDA, however, decided against approval of Contrave in February 2011, citing concerns regarding cardiovascular safety. A randomized trial has been requested by the FDA to confirm cardiovascular safety.

The endocannabinoid-receptor antagonist rimonabant held great promise in terms of weight loss and metabolic syndrome modulation, but the clinical trial program was terminated due to the issues of anxiety, depression, and suicidal ideation. Rimonabant is not approved by the FDA.

The future of pharmacologic weight loss therapies is therefore cloudy. However, there is potential for newer $5HT_{2C}$ receptor agonists, GLP-1 mimetics, as well as amylin and leptin. Liraglutide has been studied in obese individuals without T2DM and has been shown to be superior to orlistat with regard to weight loss; the prevalence of pre-diabetes was also reduced in liraglutide-treated individuals.[4] In the future, combination therapy with these agents may prove to be beneficial.

Bariatric Surgery

The generally accepted indications for bariatric surgery are (1) BMI ≥40 and (2) BMI ≥35 with comorbid conditions such as diabetes mellitus.[5] A much more controversial BMI threshold was proposed in the consensus statement from the Diabetes Surgery Summit suggesting that BMI >30 in the context of T2DM was an adequate indication for bariatric surgery.[6] Long-term success with TLC alone in these groups of patients is very uncommon. However, failure to make the necessary TLC changes after bariatric surgery can result in significant weight regain and loss of all of the therapeutic benefits of the surgery. In addition to the customary preoperative medical evaluation regarding fitness for surgery, evaluation for bariatric surgery involves comprehensive nutritional and psychological evaluation. Recovery time from surgery and surgical complications can be reduced with laparoscopic approaches when feasible. Postoperative pneumonia, deep vein thrombosis, and pulmonary embolus are of particular concern in morbidly obese subjects, and appropriate preventive measures need to be in place.

In the early postoperative period, patients are generally very pleased with the surgical results in terms of:

1. Earlier satiety
2. Decreased food cravings
3. Enhanced mobility
4. Decreased joint pain
5. Cosmetic effects of weight loss
6. Reduced severity of sleep apnea
7. Reduced venous stasis
8. Reduced gastroesophageal reflux disease (GERD)

9. Improved overall self-esteem and quality of life
10. Improved metabolic parameters in terms of:
    a. Blood glucose
    b. Lipids
    c. Uric acid
    d. Blood pressure

11. Reduced medication needs
    a. Insulin/oral anti-diabetic medications
    b. Antihypertensive agents
    c. Lipid-lowering agents

Ongoing success requires commitment to TLC regarding diet and exercise.[5]

Mechanisms of weight loss after bariatric surgery are as follows:

1. Food restriction via small pouch with resultant earlier satiety
2. Neurohumoral effects via gut peptides such as ghrelin, which reduces food cravings

Medical complications of the Roux-en-Y gastric bypass are as follows:

1. Anemia
2. Iron deficiency
3. Vitamin B12 deficiency
4. Folic acid deficiency
5. Vitamin C deficiency
6. Vitamin D deficiency with secondary hyperparathyroidism and significant bone loss on bone mineral density testing
7. Peripheral neuropathy
8. Hypoglycemia related to hyperinsulinism

Bariatric surgery is a treatment, not a cure, for T2DM. It does not address all of the pathophysiologic defects of T2DM. Overzealous surgical intervention is clearly not the answer.[7]

Plastic surgery is indicated in some patients, to include abdominoplasty, especially in the setting of recurrent intertrigo under pannus, and surgery to remove excess fat in the arms and the legs. Health care insurance coverage for such procedures can be difficult to procure.

References

1. Hollander PA, Elbein SC, Hirsch IB, et al. Role of orlistat in the treatment of obese patients with type 2 diabetes. *Diabetes Care*. 1998;21(8):1288–1294.

2. Smith SR, Weissman NJ, Anderson CM, et al. Multicenter, placebo-controlled trial of lorcaserin for weight management. *N Engl J Med*. 2010;363(3):245–256.

3. James WP, Caterson ID, Coutinho W, et al. Effect of sibutramine on cardiovascular outcomes in overweight and obese subjects. *N Engl J Med*. 2010;363(10):905–917.

4. Astrup A, Rössner S, Van Gaal L, et al. Effects of liraglutide on the treatment of obesity: A randomized, double-blind, placebo-controlled study. *Lancet*. 2009;374(9701):1606–1616.

5. Mechanick JI, Kushner RF, Sugarman HJ, et al. American Association of Clinical Endocrinologists, The Obesity Society, and American Association for Metabolic & Bariatric Surgery Medical Guidelines for the perioperative nutritional, metabolic, and non-surgical support of the bariatric surgery patient. *Endocr Pract.* 2008;14 (Suppl 1):1–83.

6. Rubino F, Kaplan LM, Schauer PR, et al. The Diabetes Surgery Summit consensus conference: Recommendations for the evaluation and use of gastrointestinal surgery to treat type 2 diabetes mellitus. *Ann Surg.* 2010;251(3):399–405.

7. Pinkney JH, Johnson AB, Gale EAM. The big fat bariatric bandwagon. *Diabetalogia.* 2010;53(9):1815–1822.

Microvascular and Macrovascular Complications of T2DM: Prevention and Treatment

Overview

The statistics on complications of DM are staggering:[1]

1. DM is the leading cause of new adult blindness in the United States.
2. DM is the leading cause of renal failure, accounting for 44% of new cases.
3. 60% to 70% of individuals with DM have neuropathy.
4. DM accounts for more than 60% of non-traumatic amputations due to a combination of neuropathy, peripheral arterial disease (PAD), and sepsis. Sensory impairment can facilitate repetitive trauma, culminating in foot ulceration. Hyperglycemia compromises wound healing, as does the ongoing trauma of walking and the tissue hypoxia related to PAD.
5. 75% of individuals with DM have HTN. HTN accelerates microvascular and macrovascular complications.
6. Adults with DM have a two- to four-fold increased death rate from CAD compared to their non-diabetic counterparts.
7. Stroke risk in individuals with DM is two- to four-fold higher than in their non-diabetic counterparts.

Albuminuria is the marker tying together microvascular and macrovascular risk. According to the Steno hypothesis,[2] albuminuria reflects widespread vascular damage and not just damage to the glomerulus. The use of ACE inhibitors or angiotensin II receptor blockers (ARBs) is effective in reducing albuminuria and preserving renal function independent of their blood pressure effect in patients with renal disease. Additionally, albuminuria has been shown to be a strong predictor of cardiovascular risk, with an 18% reduction in cardiovascular risk for every 50% reduction in albuminuria.[3]

Microvascular Complications

The clinical trial data show compelling associations between glycemic control and the microvascular complications of neuropathy, retinopathy, and nephropathy. Additionally, the earlier tight glycemic control is established, the lower the microvascular risk. Delay in instituting good glycemic control in the setting of established microvascular complications appears to prevent rapid reversal of the clinical course. This is the so-called "legacy effect" of antecedent poor glycemic control, as evidenced by long-term follow-up data from UKPDS; it is comparable to the "metabolic memory" that was seen in individuals with T1DM in the Epidemiology of Diabetes Interventions and Complications (EDIC)[4] trial, the follow-up trial to the Diabetes Control and Complications Trial (DCCT).[5] Additionally, the Steno-2 study showed that a multifactorial intervention approach over a mean treatment period of 7.8 years resulted in both microvascular and macrovascular risk reduction, including rates of death from cardiovascular and other causes.[6]

Diabetic Neuropathy

Diabetic neuropathy is subclassified as symmetric polyneuropathy, autonomic neuropathy, radiculopathy, and mononeuropathy. Symmetric polyneuropathy is the most common type, affecting initially the longest nerves of the body such that symptoms first appear in the distal toes with paresthesias and dysesthesias. On clinical exam, patients exhibit decreased sensation to pinprick, vibration sense, and Semmes-Weinstein monofilament sensation. As the neuropathy progresses, there can be loss of sensation resulting in numbness, intrinsic muscle wasting, and foot deformity, culminating in ulceration over pressure points. Later in the course, pain can develop, which patients describe as searing, stabbing pain with nocturnal intensification. Effective pharmacotherapeutic agents include tricyclic antidepressants, venlafaxine, duloxetine, gabapentin, and pregabalin. Some studies suggest that α-lipoic acid may be of some benefit, with the optimal dosing being 600 mg daily.[7] Monochromatic infrared energy therapy (anodyne therapy) in theory effects guanylate cyclase and nitrous oxide release, thereby supposedly enhancing blood flow and improving sensation. Unfortunately, a recent randomized, double-blind clinical trial proved to be negative.[8]

It is imperative to rule out other etiologies of peripheral neuropathy, such as hypothyroidism, heavy metal poisoning, and vitamin B12 deficiency. In one cross-sectional study, the prevalence of vitamin B12 deficiency, defined as a vitamin B12 level <350 pg/mL, was 22% of T2DM patients.[9] Patients with equivocal vitamin B12 levels should have methylmalonic acid levels measured. An elevated methylmalonic acid level in the setting of borderline vitamin B12 levels confirms vitamin B12 deficiency. The prevalence of vitamin B12 deficiency is higher in patients taking metformin;[10] this is most likely related to metformin-related malabsorption. Vitamin B12 deficiency is also associated with higher homocysteine levels, which may indicate increased cardiovascular risk. Curiously, the prevalence of vitamin B12 deficiency in T2DM patients appears lower in patients taking a multivitamin, suggesting some dietary deficiency rather than overt pernicious anemia. True pernicious anemia can be confirmed by positive intrinsic factor and parietal cell antibodies. Hence, not all vitamin B12 deficiency is on the basis of pernicious anemia, and it may be correctable with oral vitamin B12 supplementation.

Diabetic Retinopathy

Diabetic retinopathy is classified as background, pre-proliferative, and prolifer-ative. Annual dilated ophthalmoscopy by an ophthalmologist/optometrist is the key to early diagnosis, as visual acuity can remain stable until a catastrophic event occurs. In addition to good glycemic control, good blood pressure control is important to both the prevention/delay in the development of and progression of diabetic retinopathy, especially via ACE inhibitors. Early laser photocoagula-tion of both macular edema and hemorrhages related to proliferative retinop-athy preserves vision. Intravitreal triamcinolone is being used with increasing frequency for macular edema. Triamcinolone also has anti-angiogenic proper-ties. Bevacizumab is also being used intravitreally for the treatment of prolifer-ative diabetic retinopathy, with or without vitreous hemorrhage. Vitrectomy is reserved for situations in which other therapies have failed.

Diabetic Nephropathy

Chronic kidney disease (CKD) in diabetes is identified as microalbuminuria (≥30 mcg albumin/mg creatinine) or macroalbuminuria (≥300 mg albumin/24 hours or ≥500 mg total protein/24 hours). Creatinine clearance dictates the stages of CKD. Stage 3 CKD is characterized by a GFR of 30 to 59 mL/min and is associated with increased cardiovascular risk. Complications of renal disease include worsening HTN, hyperkalemia, hyperphosphatemia, secondary hyper-parathyroidism, hyperuricemia, progressive cardiovascular disease, renal osteo-dystrophy, anemia, and variable degrees of malnutrition/volume disorders that need to be addressed.

Microvascular complications are positively affected by:

1. HTN control, with a systolic blood pressure goal of <130 mmHg and a diastolic blood pressure goal of <80 mmHg. If nephropathy is present, the goal should be a systolic blood pressure <120 mmHg and a dia-stolic blood pressure <70 mmHg. ACE inhibitors, ARBs, and alikrenin are of particular value in the setting of nephropathy. Indeed, the UKPDS showed a 34% relative risk reduction for microvascular disease with tighter blood pressure control.[11]
2. Lipid control with statin therapy may affect microalbuminuria.
3. Smoking cessation reduces all microvascular complications.[12]
4. Antiplatelet therapy with aspirin may have an impact on early retinopa-thy progression.

Macrovascular Complications

Intensive Risk Factor Modification

Macrovascular complications of diabetes are the major contributors to morbid-ity and mortality. Intensive risk factor modification (IRFM) is recommended for all individuals with T2DM, as T2DM is a coronary risk equivalent.

Efforts to achieve macrovascular risk reduction should be aimed at:

1. LDL-C reduction
    a. Statins. LDL-C reduction to at least <100 mg/dL with statin therapy has a positive impact on MI risk reduction and stroke risk reduction.

Compelling clinical trial data suggest that a value of <70 mg/dL in high-risk patients is probably optimal.[13,14] Indeed, an LDL-C reduction of 40 mg/dL regardless of baseline LDL-C has been shown to reduce cardiovascular events.[15]

b. Ezetimibe. Can be used in statin-intolerant patients or in combination with statins to lower LDL-C. However, to date, clinical trials have failed to demonstrate cardiovascular event reduction with ezetemibe.

c. Bile acid sequestrants. Agents such as cholestyramine and colesevelam can also be used, with the latter having the additional benefit of HbA1c reduction.[16] Gastrointestinal tolerability and the timing of concomitant medications are significant issues.

d. Non-HDL-C may be superior to LDL-C in predicting coronary risk in patients with T2DM.[17]

2. Blood pressure control to systolic values <130 mmHg and diastolic values <80 mmHg. Striving for a blood pressure lower than that has failed to reduce death from cardiovascular disease or non-fatal MI, though there was a slight reduction in non-fatal stroke in the ACCORD trial.[18]

3. Smoking cessation[12]

4. Obesity management improves triglycerides and HDL-C.

5. Exercise and physical training improve survival, probably through multiple mechanisms. Several studies have conclusively demonstrated that physical fitness as measured by METS (metabolic equivalents) on a treadmill is a predictor of survival in the setting of obesity, T2DM, and coronary artery disease.[19,20]

6. Antiplatelet therapy. Primary prevention with low-dose aspirin (75–162 mg qd) is advocated for adults with DM who are at increased cardiovascular risk. This would include most men over age 50 and women over age 60 who have one or more major cardiovascular risk factors: hypertension, dyslipidemia, smoking, albuminuria, and a strong family history of premature cardiovascular disease. There is a small increased risk for hemorrhagic stroke and gastrointestinal bleeding with aspirin. Patients with risk factors such as prior gastrointestinal bleeding need to be carefully monitored. Secondary prevention with the above doses of aspirin is of course recommended for all individuals with established cardiovascular disease and diabetes. Clopidogrel is an alternative for patients with aspirin allergy.[21]

7. HDL-C issues

   a. Raising HDL-C. Raising HDL-C is prudent given the data linking low HDL-C to increased cardiovascular events. HDL may be increased by:

      i. Exercise

      ii. Niacin

      iii. Fibrates

      iv. Statin therapy, especially rosuvastatin

      v. Fish oil

vi. Moderate alcohol intake

vii. Thiazolidinedione (TZD) therapy, especially pioglitazone

b. Dysfunctional HDL-C. The absolute level of HDL-C unfortunately does not reveal the functionality of the HDL-C particle in terms of reverse cholesterol transport from macrophage foam cells, with attendant reduction in macrophage-associated inflammation. Recent *in vitro* studies suggest that attenuated HDL efflux capacity correlates inversely with carotid intima-media thickness and angiographically proven coronary artery disease.[22] Pioglitazone appears to enhance efflux capacity of the HDL particle in patients with the metabolic syndrome and low HDL-C levels.

8. Lowering triglycerides is probably prudent with regard to CAD risk, although clinical trial data are not terribly compelling. An inverse relationship exists between triglyceride and HDL-C levels. Triglyceride lowering may be achieved by:

a. Weight loss

b. Optimizing glycemic control

c. Statin therapy, especially rosuvastatin

d. Niacin

e. Fibrates

f. Fish oil

g. TZD therapy

Recent data from the ACCORD trial suggest that routine addition of fibrates to statin doses does not improve cardiac outcomes except in the setting of a low HDL-C and elevated triglycerides.[23]

9. Use of ACE inhibitors or ARBs for albuminuria regardless of blood pressure

10. Tight glycemic control: The role of tight glycemic control in preventing cardiovascular events remains controversial. Certainly the UKPDS long-term follow-up of newly diagnosed T2DM patients confirmed the benefits of tight glycemic control from the time of diagnosis of T2DM.[24,25] Intensification of glycemic control later in the course of T2DM has yielded disappointing results in the VADT,[26] ADVANCE (Action in Diabetes and Vascular Disease),[27] and ACCORD[28] trials, with either no benefit or, as seen in the ACCORD trial, increased mortality. The precise mechanism for the increased events in the ACCORD trial intensive therapy arm is unclear. However, sub-analysis revealed that the increased cardiovascular events occurred in patients with poorer baseline HbA1c randomized to intensive therapy; reported hypoglycemia *per se* did not appear to be the explanation for the increased cardiovascular events in ACCORD. However, avoidance of hypoglycemia, especially in patients with CAD, is prudent. The VADT suggested a benefit to tight glycemic control in patients with DM duration of <15 years and adverse consequences to tight glycemic control in patients with DM duration of >20 years. The results from the Steno-2 study[29] suggest that macrovascular risk reduction from intensified glycemic control may be a slow process and may

take >8 years of intensified therapy, substantially longer than the durations of the VADT, ADVANCE, and ACCORD trials.

Other

High-sensitivity C-reactive protein (hsCRP) is a marker of inflammation. CRP is produced by the liver in response to elevated cytokine production during inflammation and infection. HsCRP is an independent marker of cardiovascular risk, with individuals having elevated LDL-C and hsCRP being at highest risk. Statin therapy reduces hsCRP levels; moreover, in a study of normolipemic non-diabetic individuals with hsCRP levels ≥2.0 mg/L, rosuvastatin treatment was also associated with a dramatic reduction in cardiovascular events.[30] HsCRP levels are thus useful for stratifying cardiovascular risk. Additionally, elevated hsCRP may be a predictor of the development of T2DM.

Although increased levels of homocysteine are associated with increased cardiovascular risk, the clinical trials of homocysteine lowering have failed to show any reduction in cardiovascular events.

Screening for Coronary Artery Disease

Routine screening for CAD in asymptomatic patients remains an area of considerable controversy. Candidates for CAD screening include patients with:

1. Typical cardiac symptoms suggestive of angina
2. Atypical cardiac symptoms such as unexplained dyspnea at rest or upon exercise
3. Abnormal resting electrocardiogram (ECG)

The lack of clinical benefit of routine screening of asymptomatic individuals with T2DM was confirmed in the DIAD (Detection of Ischemia in Asymptomatic Diabetics)[31] study. Furthermore, there is emerging evidence that silent myocardial ischemia may resolve over time.[32] Screening for cardiovascular disease with electron beam computed tomography (EBCT) with a resultant coronary calcium score (CACS) score holds promise in predicting cardiovascular events in asymptomatic individuals with T2DM. An elevated CACS is a highly significant independent predictor of cardiovascular events. A doubling of CACS is associated with a 32% increase in risk of cardiovascular events. In contrast, an undetectable CACS results in mortality risks comparable to those in non-diabetic individuals.[33]

Peripheral Arterial Disease

Ankle–brachial indices (ABIs) are a good screening tool for PAD. ABIs <0.9 predict not only peripheral arterial disease but also generalized atherosclerosis and increased cardiovascular risk. ABIs can be carried out with an inexpensive handheld Doppler. The ADA consensus statement in 2003 suggested screening ABIs in the following settings:

1. All patients over age 50
2. Patients under age 50 with risk factors:
   a. DM duration >10 years
   b. HTN

   c. Dyslipidemia
   d. Smoking

Individuals with significant PAD symptoms or ABIs <0.9 should be referred for further vascular evaluation.[34]

   Caveat: Patients with significant peripheral neuropathy may not have classic symptoms of PAD.

   Management options for PAD include:

   1. Walking program
   2. Diet with decreased saturated fat plus caloric restriction in overweight/obese individuals
   3. Pentoxifylline
   4. Cilostazol
   5. Antiplatelet agents such as aspirin or clopidogrel
   6. Smoking cessation
   7. Lipid control
   8. Endovascular angioplasty and stenting
   9. Endarterectomy
   10. Surgical bypass and grafting

Cerebrovascular Disease

There are no recommendations for routine screening for cerebrovascular disease. A prospective observational study found that the risk of asymptomatic carotid stenosis >60% was highest in men with T2DM with a history of CAD (odds ratio 3.34) or an ABI <0.95 (odds ratio 3.66). Without either of these two factors the negative predictive value was 96.6%.[35] Individuals who have carotid bruits on exam should be referred for carotid duplex examination. Additionally, individuals who have transient ischemic attacks or suspicious symptoms should be referred for carotid duplex examination, and if negative, a more extensive evaluation. Atrial fibrillation is a risk factor for embolic stroke and may be managed by cardioversion, with radiofrequency ablation being reserved for patients failing repeated cardioversions. Long-term anticoagulant therapy is indicated for individuals with persistent atrial fibrillation

References

1. U.S. Department of Health and Human Services, Centers for Disease Control and Prevention. *National Diabetes Fact Sheet: National Estimates and General Information on Diabetes and Prediabetes in the United States, 2011.* Atlanta, GA.

2. Deckert T, Feldt-Rasmussen B, Borch-Johnsen K, et al. Albuminuria reflects widespread vascular damage: the Steno hypothesis. *Diabetalogia.* 1989;32(4):219–226.

3. deZeeuw D, Remuzzi G, Parving HH. Albuminuria, a therapeutic target for cardiovascular protection in type 2 diabetic patients with nephropathy. *Circulation.* 2004;110:921–927.

4. The Diabetes Control and Complications Trial/Epidemiology of Diabetes Interventions and Complications Research Group. Retinopathy and nephropathy in patients with type 1 diabetes four years after a trial of intensive therapy. *N Engl J Med.* 2000;342(6):381–389.

5. The Diabetes Control and Complications Trial Research Group. The effect of intensive treatment of diabetes on the development and progression of long-term complications in insulin-dependent diabetes mellitus. *N Engl J Med*. 1993;329(14):977–986.

6. Gaede P, Lund-Anderson H, Parving HH, et al. Effect of a multifactorial intervention on mortality in type 2 diabetes. *N Engl J Med*. 2008;358(6):580–591.

7. Ziegler D, Ametov A, Barinov A, et al. Oral treatment with α-lipoic acid improves symptomatic diabetic polyneuropathy. *Diabetes Care*. 2006;29(11):2365–2370.

8. Lavery LA, Murdoch DP, Williams J, et al. Does anodyne light therapy improve peripheral neuropathy in diabetes? A double-blind, sham-controlled, randomized trial to evaluate monochromatic infrared photoenergy. *Diabetes Care*. 2008;31(6):316–321.

9. Pflipsen MC, Oh RC, Saguil A, et al. The prevalence of vitamin B12 deficiency in patients with type 2 diabetes: A cross-sectional study. *J Am Board Fam Med*. 2009;22(5):528–534.

10. de Jager J, Kooy A, Leher P, et al. Long-term treatment with metformin in patients with type 2 diabetes and risk of vitamin B-12 deficiency: Randomized placebo controlled trial. *BMJ*. 2010; 340:c2181.

11. UK Prospective Diabetes Study (UKPDS) Group. Intensive blood-glucose control with sulphonylureas or insulin compared with conventional treatment and risk of complications in patients with type 2 diabetes (UIPDS 33). *Lancet*. 1998;352(9131):837–853.

12. American Diabetes Association. Smoking and diabetes. *Diabetes Care*. 2004;27(Suppl 1):S74-S75.

13. Colhoun HM, Betteridge DJ, Durrington PN, et al. Primary prevention of cardiovascular disease with atorvastatin in type 2 diabetes in the Collaborative Atorvastatin Diabetes Study (CARDS): Multicentre randomized placebo-controlled trial. *Lancet*. 2004;364(9435):685–696.

14. Collins R, Armitage J, Parish S, et al. MRC/BHF heart protection study of cholesterol-lowering with simvastatin in 5963 people with diabetes: A randomized placebo-controlled trial. *Lancet*. 2003;361(9324):2005–2016.

15. Cholesterol Treatment Trialists' (CTT) Collaborators. Efficacy of cholesterol-lowering therapy in 18, 686 people with diabetes in 14 randomised trials of statins: A meta-analysis. *Lancet*. 2008;371(9607):117–125.

16. Fonseca VA, Rosenstock J, Wang AC. Colesevelam HCL improves glycemic control and reduces LDL cholesterol in patients with inadequately controlled type 2 diabetes on sulfonylurea-based therapy. *Diabetes Care*. 2008;31(8):1479–1481.

17. Liu J, Sempos CT, Donahue RP, et al. Non-high density lipoprotein and very-low density lipoprotein cholesterol and their risk predictive values in coronary heart disease. *Am J Cardiol*. 2006;98(10):1363–1368.

18. The ACCORD Study Group. Effects of intensive blood-pressure control in type 2 diabetes mellitus. *N Engl J Med*. 2010;362(17):1575–1585.

19. Myers J, Prakash M, Froelicher V, et al. Exercise capacity and mortality among men referred for exercise testing. *N Engl J Med*. 2002;346(11):763–801.

20. Gulati M, Pandey DK, Arnsdorf MF, et al. Exercise capacity and the risk of death in women: The St. James Women Take Heart project. *Circulation*. 2003;108(13):1554–1559.

21. Pignone M, Alberts MJ, Colwell JA, et al. Aspirin for primary prevention of cardiovascular events in people with diabetes. A position statement of the American Diabetes Association, a scientific statement of the American Heart Association, and an expert consensus document of the American College of Cardiology Foundation. *Diabetes Care*. 2010;33(6):1395–1402.

22. Khera AV, Cuchel M, de la Llero-Moya M, et al. Cholesterol efflux capacity, high-density lipoprotein function, and atherosclerosis. *N Engl J Med*. 2011;364(2):127–135.

23. The ACCORD Study Group. Effects of combination lipid therapy in type 2 diabetes mellitus. *N Engl J Med*. 2010;362(17):1563–1574.

24. Holman RR, Paul SK, Bethal MA, et al. 10-year follow-up of intensive glucose control in type 2 diabetes. *N Engl J Med*. 2008;359(15):1577–1589.

25. Chalmers J, Cooper ME. UKPDS and the legacy effect. *N Engl J Med*. 2008;359(15):1618–1620.

26. Duckworth W, Abraira C, Moritz T, et al. Glucose control and vascular complication in veterans with type 2 diabetes. *N Engl J Med*. 2009;360(2):129–139.

27. The ADVANCE Collaborative Group. Intensive blood glucose control and vascular outcomes in patiens with type 2 diabetes. *N Engl J Med*. 2008;360(24):2503–2515.

28. The Action to Control Cardiovascular Risk in Diabetes Study Group. Effect of intensive glucose lowering in type 2 diabetes. *N Engl J Med*. 2008;358(24):2545–2559.

29. Gaede P, Lund-Anderson H, Parving HH, et al. Effect of a multifactorial intervention on mortality in type 2 diabetes. *N Engl J Med*. 2008;358(6):580–591.

30. Ridker PM, Danielson E, Fonseca FAH, et al. for the JUPITER Study Group. Rosuvastatin to prevent vascular events in men and women with elevated C-reactive protein. *N Engl J Med*. 2008;359(21):2195–2207.

31. Young LH, Wackers FJ, Chyun DA, et al. for the DIAD Investigators. Cardiac outcomes after screening for asymptomatic coronary artery disease in patients with type 2 diabetes: The DIAD study. *JAMA*. 2009;301(15):1547–1555.

32. Wackers FJ, Chyun DA, Young LH, et al. Resolution of asymptomatic myocardial ischemia in patients with type 2 diabetes mellitus in the DIAD study. *Diabetes Care*. 2007;30(11):2892–2898.

33. Elkeles RS, Godsland IF, Feher MD, et al. Coronary calcium measurement improves prediction of cardiovascular events in asymptomatic patients with type 2 diabetes: the PREDICT study. *Eur Heart J*. 2008;29(18):2244–2251.

34. American Diabetes Association. Peripheral arterial disease in people with diabetes (Consensus Statement). *Diabetes Care*. 2003;26(12):3333–3341.

35. Lacroix P, Aboyans V, Criqui MH, et al. Type-2 diabetes and carotid stenosis: A proposal for a screening strategy in asymptomatic patients. *Vasc Med*. 2006;11(2):93–99.

Chapter 7

Common Comorbidities of T2DM and Obesity

Obstructive Sleep Apnea

Obstructive sleep apnea (OSA) is a common disorder occurring in the setting of T2DM and obesity, with a prevalence as high as 86% being reported in one study.[1] Although the majority of these patients are obese, approximately 30% are not.[2] The clinical clues to OSA include:

1. Excess snoring
2. Witnessed apneic spells
3. Morning or nighttime headaches
4. Daytime hypersomnolence or falling asleep readily
5. Chronic fatigue
6. Restless sleep
7. High waist circumference/high BMI

Silent nocturnal coronary ischemia associated with O_2 desaturation is of major concern. Additionally, OSA is associated with insulin resistance, visceral adiposity, and inflammation.[3] Recent data on OSA in children demonstrates a negative impact on learning and academic performance.[4] This, of course, has life-long sequelae.

The adverse effects of OSA are well recognized, but there is growing awareness that poor sleep hygiene may have adverse effects other than fatigue.

Insufficient sleep may:[5,6]

1. Reduce an individual's ability to lose weight on a hypocaloric diet
2. Raise ghrelin levels
3. Promote feelings of hunger
4. Lower leptin levels and decrease satiety

Therefore, attention to proper sleep hygiene is important for all individuals, regardless of BMI.

The chronic fatigue and daytime hypersomnolence associated with OSA presents a major obstacle to TLC in the patient with T2DM and may be the explanation for apparent non-adherence, or perhaps more appropriately the inability to adhere to the prescribed regimen.

Referral to a sleep specialist and a formal sleep study will confirm the diagnosis. After a period of appropriate continuous positive airway pressure (C-PAP) or biphasic airway pressure (Bi-PAP) therapy with optimization of pressures,

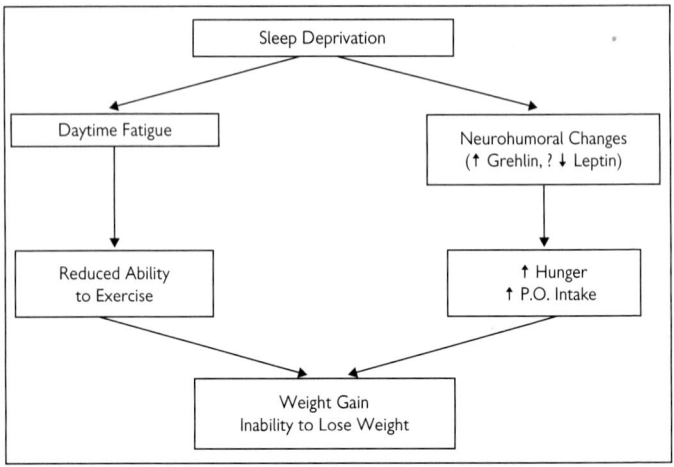

Figure 7.1 Sleep deprivation

patients generally report a dramatic improvement in overall well-being and ability to work on diet and exercise. Residual daytime hypersomnolence may warrant the prescribing of modafinil (Provigil) or armodafinil (Nuvigil).

Male Hypogonadism, T2DM, and Obesity

The prevalence of hypogonadism in men with T2DM is double that of the general population and is compounded by obesity, hypertension, dyslipidemia, and advancing age.[7] One study suggested that the true prevalence was in excess of 50% of men with T2DM.[8] Common symptoms of hypogonadism include:

1. Fatigue
2. Muscle weakness
3. Erectile dysfunction
4. Loss of libido
5. Loss of lean body mass
6. Increased body fat
7. Decreased body and facial hair
8. Unexplained anemia
9. Decreased physical endurance
10. Decreased bone mass

Frequently these symptoms are overlooked or attributed to aging or the diabetes *per se*.

After an initial early-morning testosterone level has been found to be low, to distinguish primary hypogonadism from secondary hypogonadism, it is important to have further evaluation done in the fasting state (8 a.m.) of the following hormones: follicle-stimulating hormone (FSH), luteinizing hormone (LH), pro-lactin, and a repeat total testosterone. Elevated FSH and LH levels would indicate secondary hypogonadism. If the prolactin level is elevated, this may be related to a pituitary neoplasm, medications such as metoclopramide, hypothyroidism, or renal insufficiency. Subnormal FSH and LH levels would warrant evaluation for a pituitary neoplasm.

Once the decision to initiate androgen replacement therapy has been made, confirmation of a normal baseline prostate-specific antigen (PSA) level is critical. Androgen replacement therapy with a view to restoring testosterone levels to the mid-normal range can be accomplished with topical preparations, patches, or depot injections and can have a dramatic effect on the features of hypogonadism. It is important to stress to patients that testosterone replacement therapy is not just for sexual function. Concerns about testosterone replacement therapy in the setting of OSA revolve around a study in which supraphysiologic testosterone replacement worsened sleep apnea.[9] However, there is no evidence that physiologic testosterone replacement to the mid-normal range has any negative effect on sleep apnea—rather, there is a positive effect. Furthermore, correction of low testosterone levels has been found to have a positive impact on risk of both T2DM and CAD.[7,8,10,11] Ongoing assessment of PSA is obviously necessary for early detection of possible prostate cancer.

Hypovitaminosis D and T2DM

Low levels of vitamin D are very prevalent in residents of the northern latitudes due to limited sun exposure. Even residents of equatorial and southern latitudes can have low levels for the same reasons. Individuals with T2DM and obesity also tend to have low vitamin D levels. The ramification of this is not simply limited to decreased bone health, which is due in part to varying degrees of secondary hyperparathyroidism. Severe vitamin D deficiency predicts increased all-cause and cardiovascular mortality independent of cardiovascular risk factors and micro- or macroalbuminuria. The impact of vitamin D replacement on mortality is yet to be determined.[12] Additionally, a cross-sectional study showed that low levels of vitamin D are associated with beta-cell dysfunction and insulin resistance in subjects at risk for T2DM; the impact of vitamin D replacement in this scenario is speculative.[13]

The 2010 Institute of Medicine report generated considerable controversy in regard to the optimal vitamin D level for the general population, not to mention the defining of the safe level of supplementation.[14] The data regarding skeletal health suggest a 25-hydroxy vitamin D level of 20 ng/mL to be adequate, with a safe, supplemented upper limit of 50 ng/mL. The extraskeletal associations of vitamin D deficiency include diabetes, autoimmune disorders, cardiovascular disease, and cancer. The optimal level of 25-hydroxy vitamin D for these extraskeletal associations remains unknown. Further studies are clearly warranted.

Hypoglycemia

Absolute Hypoglycemia

The counter-regulatory response to hypoglycemia is generally activated with ambient blood glucose levels <70 mg/dL in individuals without diabetes. In individuals with diabetes, adrenergic symptoms (tremors, tachycardia, anxiety, agitation) and cholinergic symptoms (excess sweating and hunger) can arise in roughly the range of 65 to 70 mg/dL. Neuroglycopenic symptoms (behavior changes that may mimic alcohol excess, mental confusion, psychomotor retardation) typically present at a lower glycemic threshold (~50–55 mg/dL).[15] Severe hypoglycemia is defined as a low blood glucose value that cannot be self-treated by the individual and requires the assistance of another individual. This assistance can be with oral feeding or glucagon administration or via IV dextrose administered by a health care professional. Severe hypoglycemia can result in seizures, coma, and brain death, although this is rare. Despite popular belief, fatal cases of hypoglycemia are not limited to individuals with T1DM.[16] Fatal cases of sulfonylurea-associated hypoglycemia have also been recorded.[17]

Hypoglycemia is the rate-limiting step in the intensity to which DM is managed.

The prevalence of hypoglycemia in patients with T2DM is high. Continuous glucose monitoring studies have suggested that many patients with T2DM have unrecognized hypoglycemia. One study suggested that the prevalence was in excess of 40%, which is clearly quite disturbing; over 70% of the events occurred at night.[18] This is especially worrisome given that the counter-regulatory hormonal response to hypoglycemia is blunted at night. Emergency room visits for hypoglycemia reveal that 44% of the events occur in adults over the age of 65 years, with most of these individuals having T2DM.[19]

Risk factors for hypoglycemia include:

1. Advanced age with associated poor symptom recognition
2. Long duration of diabetes
3. Blunted awareness of hypoglycemia
4. Missed meals, delayed meals, or reduced carbohydrate intake
5. Uncompensated physical activity
6. Insulin therapy, especially with multiple daily insulin injections and improper matching of insulin to carbohydrate intake and/or excess basal insulin
7. Secretagogue therapy with sulfonylureas
8. Excess self-dosing of secretagogues or insulin
9. Near-normal HbA1c values in the context of insulin or secretagogue therapy

The adverse effects of hypoglycemia on the heart have received a lot of attention recently in the light of the surprising results of the ACCORD trial in terms of increased mortality associated with intensive therapy of T2DM.[20] Although hypoglycemia could not be determined to be the culprit, it was nonetheless given a lot of consideration. Hypoglycemia is of particular concern in individuals with underlying CAD due to the following (Fig. 7.2):

1. Q-T prolongation with attendant arrhythmia risk
2. Sympathetic activation with arrhythmia risk

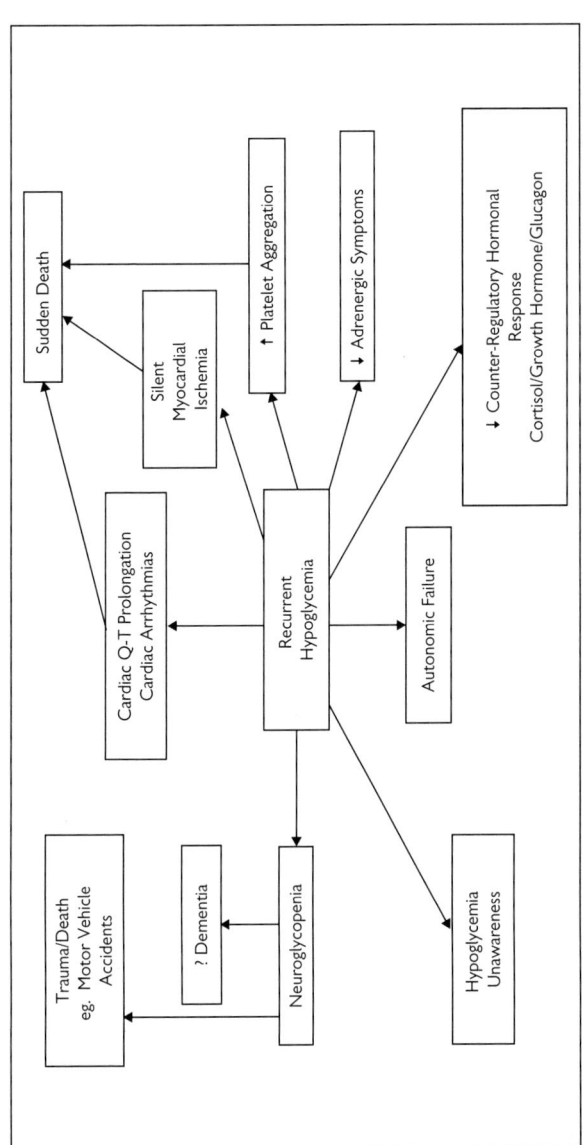

Figure 7.2 Sequelae of recurrent hypoglycemia

3. Increased platelet aggregation and thrombotic risk
4. Potential for sudden death

A recent clinical trial involving 72-hour simultaneous Holter monitoring and continuous glucose monitoring revealed that symptomatic and asymptomatic hypoglycemia was associated with chest pain and ECG abnormalities in individuals with DM and underlying CAD.[21] This is clearly of clinical concern. Abolition of ischemic preconditioning has been a longstanding issue with regard to sulfonylurea therapy. The UKPDS trial, however, failed to show any increased cardiovascular risk associated with the prescription of sulfonylureas.[22]

Dementia and hypoglycemia may have an associative relationship. A Kaiser Permanente observational study raised the possibility that repeated severe hypoglycemia may be a significant risk factor for future dementia.[23] This was the first study to suggest such a relationship, as most prior studies have failed to show significant cognitive compromise from hypoglycemia unless hypoglycemia was extremely prolonged and associated with seizure activity. It is plausible that many of the individuals in the Kaiser Permanente study had some cognitive compromise prior to a formal diagnosis of dementia, which predisposed them to hypoglycemia in the setting of insulin and sulfonylurea therapy.

The hypoglycemia associated with islet hyperplasia, islet hypertrophy, and nesidioblastosis is generally postprandial, although the occasional patient may present with fasting hypoglycemia. Increased attention was drawn to this entity by the Mayo Clinic report of six patients with this disorder following Roux-en-Y gastric bypass surgery.[24] Only one of the patients proved to have an insulinoma, with the other five patients having islet hypertrophy/hyperplasia, possibly on the basis of augmented GLP-1 secretion following the bypass surgery. The patient with the insulinoma was managed with a spleen-preserving distal pancreatectomy. Given the increasing numbers of patients undergoing Roux-en-Y gastric bypass, clinicians need to be alerted to this entity and its management. In the majority of cases, individuals post-gastric bypass can be managed as outlined in the section that follows on reactive hypoglycemia.

Hypoglycemia Unawareness

Poor awareness for hypoglycemia is especially prevalent among individuals who have had repeated episodes of hypoglycemia and appear to tolerate much lower blood glucose levels without appropriate adrenergic/cholinergic symptomatology. In many instances, the only symptom is neuroglycopenia and loss of consciousness. Hypoglycemia unawareness is more common in insulin-treated individuals but can occur in individuals with T2DM treated with sulfonylureas. The probable underlying pathophysiology is an increase in blood glucose transporters at the level of the blood–brain barrier in response to repeated hypoglycemia, thereby allowing the brain to continue to function at lower ambient blood glucose levels. Additionally, the normal counter-regulatory response is blunted in these individuals. Hypoglycemia unawareness can be reversed with the elimination of all hypoglycemia; this has been best demonstrated in individuals with T1DM. However, the same principles probably apply to insulin-treated insulinopenic T2DM individuals. After all hypoglycemia has been eliminated for a period of several weeks, gradual restoration of hypoglycemia awareness will occur. The counter-regulatory hormonal response to hypoglycemia also improves. This is clearly a major safety issue with regard to insulin therapy.

Reactive Hypoglycemia

Reactive hypoglycemia in a non-diabetic individual generally occurs 2 to 4 hours postprandially with the presence of dominant adrenergic symptoms consisting of tremors, tachycardia, excess sweating, and variable degrees of fatigue. Reactive hypoglycemia is confirmed by the following triad:

1. Symptoms of hypoglycemia as above
2. A documented blood glucose level in the hypoglycemic range at the time concurrent with the individual's symptoms
3. Prompt resolution of the symptoms within 10 minutes of consumption of simple carbohydrate

Many individuals present with a self-diagnosis of hypoglycemia, but the majority of them fail to meet the above criteria. True reactive hypoglycemia reflects disordered insulin secretion, such that the individual had (1) a delayed early insulin response to the ingestion of simple carbohydrate and (2) later hypersecretion of insulin, resulting in varying degrees of hypoglycemia. True reactive hypoglycemia is recognized as a forerunner of future overt T2DM. Many affected individuals have a positive family history of T2DM. In clinical practice, the best way to diagnose this condition is via home blood glucose monitoring when the individual is symptomatic.

Management of reactive hypoglycemia involves the avoidance of consuming simple carbohydrates and the consumption of a diet high in fiber and low-glycemic-index carbohydrates. If the individual is obese, appropriate caloric restriction is also appropriate. Optimization of physical fitness is also important with regard to optimization of insulin sensitivity to try to blunt the late postprandial insulin response. There is no FDA-approved pharmacotherapy for reactive hypoglycemia, but off-label use of the alpha-glucosidase inhibitors acarbose and miglitol may be of help in select individuals. Additionally, the off-label use of metformin may be of value for its insulin sensitization properties. All patients with reactive hypoglycemia should be monitored for the development of overt T2DM. Patients should also be evaluated for the presence of other elements of the metabolic syndrome and should be managed accordingly.

Hyperinsulinemic Fasting Hypoglycemia in the Non-diabetic Individual

Insulinoma is a rare cause of fasting hypoglycemia; it is generally not associated with obesity. These individuals present with fasting hypoglycemia and neuroglycopenic symptoms. The occasional patient may present with postprandial hypoglycemia. The diagnostic test for insulinoma is a 72-hour fast; an inappropriate insulin:glucose ratio is generally found early on. A triple-phase CT scan can be used for localization in addition to a selective arterial calcium stimulation test. Intraoperative palpation of the pancreas and intraoperative ultrasonography can be helpful in localization.

Factitious Hypoglycemia

The true incidence of factitious hypoglycemia is unknown; it certainly provides a significant challenge to the clinician. Surreptitious use of insulin and sulfonylureas in non-diabetic individuals will result in hypoglycemia. Frequently, these individuals have access to sulfonylureas or insulin via a family member or employment situation in health care. Indeed, the first associated factitious hypoglycemia was described in 1944 and involved a nurse. Surreptitious insulin use in a non-diabetic will result in suppressed C-peptide and pro-insulin levels in the setting of hypoglycemia. Surreptitious sulfonylurea use will result in elevated C-peptide and pro-insulin levels in the context of elevated plasma or urine sulfonylurea levels.

In insulin-treated individuals, intentional insulin overdose can be seen in the setting of eating disorders and other mental illnesses. This can occur both in the home setting and the hospital setting, where patients or their family members may surreptitiously inject extra insulin. This scenario is a lot more difficult to document and should always be considered in the setting of unexplained hypoglycemia in an insulin-treated individual. Sulfonylurea excess can occur, especially in older individuals, related to prescribing errors, prescription filling errors, or accidental overdosing. Therefore, review of the individual's medication list and especially medication containers frequently reveals the error.

Asymptomatic Hyperuricemia

Elevated uric acid levels have many clinical associations outside of clinical gout and uric acid kidney stone disease, as outlined in Table 7.1. However, associations are certainly not causality.[25]

Uric acid levels have been rising as people migrate to urban environments from their native rural backgrounds. Increased intakes of fructose, purine-rich fatty meats, and alcohol are associated with increased uric acid levels. Uric acid levels tend to be lower in women, probably on the basis of the uricosuric effect of estrogen. This could theoretically positively modulate cardiovascular risk in

Table 7.1 Associations of Asymptomatic Hyperuricemia
Cerebrovascular disease/dementia
Coronary artery disease
Diabetes mellitus
Elevated high-sensitivity CRP
Endothelial dysfunction
Hypertension
Metabolic syndrome/insulin resistance
Microalbuminuria
Obesity
Obstructive sleep apnea
Renal disease

premenopausal women. There is certainly a strong association with hyperuricemia and the metabolic syndrome; however, some recent data suggest that there is an 80% excess risk of the development of HTN over 6 years among men with asymptomatic hyperuricemia without the metabolic syndrome.[26] Additionally, in the second Nurses' Health Study, baseline uric acid levels correlated with insulin sensitivity and the risk of future hypertension.[27] A recent study in Chinese individuals showed a modest positive association between uric acid levels and future T2DM during a 9-year follow-up period.[28] Finally, a recent randomized clinical trial showed a beneficial effect of allopurinol treatment on blood pressure levels in adolescents with asymptomatic hyperuricemia and newly diagnosed HTN. However, this was a short-term 4-week study with 30% of the participants meeting the criteria for the metabolic syndrome and 70% of them being obese. In this study, the blood pressure normalized in 86% of the individuals when the uric acid level was normalized to less than 5 mg/dL.[29] This provocative study raises the question as to whether hyperuricemia may actually be important in the pathogenesis of HTN.

Animal studies in rats with uricase inhibition and elevated uric acid levels have shown the development of HTN; amelioration of the HTN results with the use of xanthine oxidase inhibitors and uricosuric agents.[30] Additionally, the hyperuricemia induced microvascular changes in the kidney similar to those seen in hypertensive nephrosclerosis. Once these lesions were induced, the animals needed to maintain a low-salt diet to maintain blood pressure in the normal range, thereby suggesting the induction of a salt-sensitive state.[31]

Hyperuricemia is associated with decreased endothelial nitric oxide production, vascular smooth muscle cell proliferation, increased oxidative stress, activation of the local renin-angiotensin system, elevated intraglomerular pressure, and sodium retention. Interestingly, allopurinol has been shown to decrease the rate of progression in renal disease in patients with stage III chronic kidney disease.[32] Additionally, discontinuing allopurinol in patients with chronic kidney disease has been shown to be associated with worsening hypertension and acceleration of the rate of progression of renal disease.[33]

All of the aforementioned data are certainly provocative with regard to the role of uric acid elevation in vascular and renal disease. However, the data are not strong enough to support the routine use of uric acid-lowering agents in patients with asymptomatic hyperuricemia. Currently urate-lowering therapy is not indicated outside of gout and uric acid kidney stone disease.[34]

References

1. Foster GD, Sanders MH, Millman R, et al. Obstructive sleep apnea among obese patients with type 2 diabetes. *Diabetes Care*. 2009;32(6):1017–1019.

2. Wolk R, Shamsuzzaman AS, Somers VK. Obesity, sleep apnea, and hypertension. *Hypertension*. 2006;42(1):1067–1074.

3. Trakada G, Chrousos G, Pejovic S, et al. Sleep apnea and its association with the stress system, inflammation, insulin resistance and visceral obesity. *Sleep Med Clin*. 2007;2(2):11–16.

4. Beebe DW, Ris M, Kramer M, et al. The association between sleep-disordered breathing, academic grades, and neurobehavioral function among overweight subjects during middle to late childhood. *J Sleep Sleep Disorders Res.* 2010;33 (Suppl 1): Abstract 0980, A327.

5. Schmid SM, Hallschmid M, Jauch-Chara K, et al. A single night of sleep deprivation increases ghrelin levels and feelings of hunger in normal-weight healthy men. *J Sleep Res.* 2008;17(3):331–334.

6. Nedeltcheva AV, Kildus JM, Imperial J, et al. Insufficient sleep undermines dietary efforts to reduce adiposity. *Ann Intern Med.* 2010;153(7):435–441.

7. Mulligan T, Frick MF, Zuraw QC, et al. Prevalence of hypogonadism in males aged at least 45 years: The HIM study. *Int J Clin Pract.* 2006;60(7):762–769.

8. Dhindsa S, Prabhakar S, Sethi M, et al. Frequent occurrence of hypogonadtropic hypogonadism in type 2 diabetes. *J Clin Endocrinol Metab.* 2004; 89(11): 5432–5468.

9. Liu PY, Yee B, Wishart SM, et al. The short-term effects of high-dose testosterone on sleep, breathing, and function in older men. *J Clin Endocrinol Metab.* 2003;88(8):3605–3613.

10. Makhsida N, Shah I, Yan G, et al. Hypogonadism and metabolic syndrome: Implications for testosterone therapy. *J Urol.* 2005;174(3):827–834.

11. Potenza M, Shimsi M. Male hypogonadism: The unrecognized cardiovascular risk factor. *J Clin Lipid.* 2007;2(2):71–78.

12. Joergensen C, Gall M, Schmedes A, et al. Vitamin D levels and mortality in type 2 diabetes. *Diabetes Care.* 2010;33(10):2238–2243.

13. Kayaniyil S, Vieth R, Retnakaran R, et al. Association of vitamin D with insulin resistance and ß-cell function in subjects at risk for type 2 diabetes. *Diabetes Care.* 2010;33(6):1379–1381.

14. Committee to Review Dietary References Intakes for Vitamin D and Calcium, Food and Nutrition Board. Institute of Medicine of the National Academies. Dietary reference intakes: Calcium and vitamin D (2011). The National Academies Press; Washington, D. C. Available on line at http://books.nap.edu/openbook.php?record_id=13050.

15. Cryer PE, Davis SN, Shamoon H. Hypoglycemia in diabetes. *Diabetes Care.* 2003;26(6):1902–1912.

16. Cryer PE. Mechanisms of sympathoadrenal failure and hypoglycemia in diabetes. *J Clin Invest.* 2006;116(6):1470–1473.

17. Shorr RI, Ray WA, Daugherty JR, et al. Incidence and risk factors for serious hypoglycemia in older persons using insulin or sulfonylureas. *Arch Intern Med.* 1997;157(15):1681–1686.

18. Chico A, Vidal-Rios P, Subirà M, et al. The continuous glucose monitoring system is useful for detecting unrecognized hypoglycemias in patients with type 1 and type 2 diabetes but is not better than frequent capillary glucose measurements for improving metabolic control. *Diabetes Care.* 2003;26(4):1153–1157.

19. Ginde AA, Espinola JA, Camargo CA. Trends and disparities in U.S. emergency department visits for hypoglycemia, 1993–1995. *Diabetes Care.* 2008;31(3): 511–513.

20. The Action to Control Cardiovascular Risk in Diabetes Study Group. Effect of intensive glucose lowering in type 2 diabetes. *N Engl J Med.* 2008;358(24):2545–2559.

21. Desouza C, Salazar H, Cheong B, et al. Association of hypoglycemia and cardiac ischemia. *Diabetes Care.* 2003;26(5):1485–1489.

22. UK Prospective Diabetes Study (UKPDS) Group. Intensive blood-glucose control with sulphonylureas or insulin compared with conventional treatment and risk of complications in patients with type 2 diabetes. (UKPDS 33). *Lancet.* 1998;352(9131):837–853.

23. Whitmer RA, Karter AJ, Yaffe K, et al. Hypoglycemic episodes and risk of dementia in older patients with type 2 diabetes mellitus. *JAMA.* 2009;301(15):1565–1572.

24. Service GJ, Thompson GB, Service FJ, et al. Hyperinsulinemic hypoglycemia with nesidioblastosis after gastric-bypass surgery. *N Engl J Med.* 2005; 353(3):249–254.

25. Feig DI, Kang D-H, Johnson RJ. Uric acid and cardiovascular risk. *N Engl J Med.* 2008;359(17):1811–1821.

26. Krishnan E, Kwoh CK, Schumacher R, et al. Hyperuricemia and incidence of hypertension among men without metabolic syndrome. *Hypertension.* 2007;49(2):298–303.

27. Forman JP, Choi H, Curhan GC. Uric acid and insulin sensitivity and risk of incident hypertension. *Arch Intern Med.* 2009;169(2):155–162.

28. Chien K-L, Chen M-F, Hsu H-C, et al. Plasma uric acid and the risk of type 2 diabetes in a Chinese community. *Clin Chem.* 2008;54(2):310–316.

29. Feig DI, Solestky B, Johnson RJ. Effect of allopurinol on blood pressure of adolescents with newly diagnosed essential hypertension: A randomized trial. *JAMA.* 2008;300(8):924–932.

30. Mazzali M, Hughes J, Kim Y-G, et al. Elevated uric acid increases blood pressure in the rat by a novel crystal-independent mechanism. *Hypertension.* 2001;38(5):1101–1106.

31. Franco M, Tapia E, Santamaria J, et al. Renal cortical vasoconstriction contributes to development of salt-sensitive hypertension after angiotensin II exposure. *J Am Soc Nephrol.* 2001;12(11):2263–2271.

32. Siu Y-P, Leung KT, Tong MK, et al. Use of allopurinol in slowing the progression of renal disease through its ability to lower serum uric acid level. *Am J Kidney Dis.* 2006;47(1):51–59.

33. Talaat KM, El-Sheikh AR. The effect of mild hyperuricemia on urinary transforming growth factor beta and the progression of chronic kidney disease. *Am J Nephrol.* 2007;27(5):435–440.

34. Edwards NL. The role of hyperurciemia and gout in kidney and cardiovascular disease. *Cleveland Clinic J Med.* 2008;75(5):S13-S16.

Chapter 8

Special Situations and T2DM

Cancer, T2DM, and Obesity

A risk between obesity and several cancers has long been established. The compounding effect of T2DM has been a matter of controversy. A recent consensus report suggested a true increase in several cancers, including postmenopausal breast cancer, endometrial cancer, colorectal cancer, hepatocellular cancer, pancreatic cancer, and non-Hodgkin's lymphoma.[1] Additionally, the presence of DM in these cancers increases both the short-term and long-term mortality.

The roles of chronic hyperglycemia, hyperinsulinemia, elevated BMI, chronic inflammation, and mode of diabetes treatment[2] need to be elucidated regarding cancer risk. In terms of diabetes treatment modality, concern was raised that insulin glargine might be associated with an increased risk of malignancy, based largely on administrative databases rather than randomized clinical trials. This provoked concern for patients and physicians alike; however, prescribing associations do not amount to causality.[3] Curiously, metformin prescription has been associated with decreased cancer risk.[4] This may be accounted for by the fact that metformin is generally prescribed earlier in the course of T2DM, or perhaps by other biologic effects apart from insulin sensitization.

Psychosocial Issues in T2DM and Obesity

Obesity and T2DM are more challenging disorders to manage due to the significant element of behavioral changes versus just medication adherence, such as in hypothyroidism as an example. The multinational DAWN study, which addressed barriers to improved diabetes management, reached the following conclusions:[5]

1. 41% of patients reported poor psychological well-being based on the WHO-5 well-being index and a history of recent treatment for psychological problems.
2. Regimen adherence problems involving diet, exercise, medication, home blood glucose monitoring, and appointment keeping were very prevalent. Only 39% of T2DM patients achieved complete success in at least two thirds of their self-care domains. Diet and exercise proved to be the most problematic domains.

Depression is common among individuals with chronic illnesses, especially in the setting of concurrent obesity, and most studies in T2DM reveal a prevalence in excess of 25%. Depression may be compounded by various psychosocial stressors, including employment issues, health insurance, and family dynamics. These individuals are thus incapable of complying with a diet and exercise program and their illness may spiral out of control until the depression is addressed.[6]

The efficacy of standard antidepressant regimen is comparable in individuals with T2DM and their non-diabetic counterparts. For optimal outcomes, pharmacotherapy is best complemented by ongoing behavior therapy.

Eating disorders such as anorexia and bulimia must be looked for in individuals with a lot of unexplained glucose lability.[7] Hypoglycemia can ensue if patients taking meal-time insulin later induce emesis to control weight. Diabulimia is a condition in T1DM patients in which individuals engage in intentional caloric purging via glycosuria induced by deliberate insulin dose reduction/elimination with resultant hyperglycemia. Eating-disordered T2DM patients may also use this approach to control weight.

A careful clinical history, which may include depression inventories such as the Beck Depression Inventory and Hamilton Depression Scale, is needed to unearth these disorders. Appropriate pharmacotherapy and psychotherapy can dramatically improve the plight of these individuals and help restore glycemia.

Secondary (Atypical) Antipsychotic Agents and T2DM

The use of second-generation (atypical) antipsychotics has been associated with new-onset T2DM and in some cases overt diabetic ketoacidosis and mortality. Individuals with schizophrenia have a 2.7-fold increased mortality from diabetes and a 2.3-fold increased mortality from cardiovascular disease. Atypical antipsychotics appear to increase insulin resistance and promote weight gain through uncertain mechanisms, with the highest prevalence appearing with clozapine and olanzapine.[8]

Frequently, patients with schizophrenia and/or bipolar disorder have psychiatrists as their only physician. Psychiatrists therefore must be vigilant with regard to monitoring glucose parameters in individuals treated with atypical antipsychotics, especially those with risk factors for T2DM such as obesity and/or a positive family history of T2DM.[9] Should an individual treated with a second-generation agent gain ≥5% of his or her initial weight, consideration should be given to switching to a different second-generation agent. Likewise, individuals who experience worsening glycemia or dyslipidemia should be switched to an alternative second-generation agent.[8]

Management of T2DM in patients treated with antipsychotic should be along conventional lines, including TLC plus metformin, assuming no contraindications

Pregnancy

T2DM

T2DM may antedate pregnancy or be diagnosed early in the pregnancy at the patient's first prenatal visit, in contradistinction to true gestational diabetes mellitus (GDM), for which screening takes place traditionally at 24 weeks' gestation. Tight glycemic control prior to conception in patients with established diabetes is critical to minimizing the risk of congenital abnormalities. Frequently, patients newly diagnosed with T2DM in pregnancy are individuals who have actually had undiagnosed DM for several years. Hence, they need to be evaluated for microvascular and macrovascular complications that might be problematic in pregnancy, such as retinopathy, nephropathy, and cardiovascular disease. ACE inhibitors, ARBs, statins, and most non-insulin therapies will need to be discontinued, ideally before conception but certainly immediately upon confirmation of pregnancy.[10]

Glycemic goals in pregnancy are tighter than in the non-pregnant state because glucose levels are lower in normal pregnancy. These goals are preprandial blood glucose levels <90 mg/dL and 2-hour postprandial blood glucose levels <120 mg/dL. Macrosomia results largely from failure to meet the 2-hour postprandial glycemic goals.

When dietary changes fail to achieve goal glucose levels, the only recommended pharmacotherapeutic agent is insulin therapy. In patients with T2DM and polycystic ovarian syndrome PCOS who experience recurrent spontaneous abortions, the use of metformin throughout the pregnancy has been associated with a reduced risk of fetal loss. Various insulin regimens have been advocated in pregnancy, with some dispute regarding the use of analog insulins. Endogenous maternal insulin does not cross the placenta, and there is no evidence that exogenous insulin crosses the placenta. Given that analog insulins have more predictable kinetics and are associated with less hypoglycemia, we prefer their use, especially when seeking the super-strict glycemic goals of pregnancy. Some patients may initially require only basal insulin. As postprandial hyperglycemia develops, RAA insulin is administered before meals. Frequently, the first meal of the day requiring RAA is the evening meal, as it usually contains the highest carbohydrate composition of the day. RAA can then be added to other meals/snacks pending postprandial hyperglycemia. Full basal-bolus therapy may be required, especially in (1) leaner individuals, (2) more insulin-resistant individuals, and (3) those with advancing pregnancy. Some centers use alternative regimens akin to those used in T2DM. Rare centers still use human regular insulin and human NPH insulin; however, postprandial glycemic goals are next to impossible to achieve with these regimens without unacceptable hypoglycemia.[10]

Insulin requirements can increase dramatically in pregnancy because of escalating insulin resistance, largely due to rising human placental lactogen (HPL) levels. Close follow-up is therefore needed to maintain patients at goal glycemic levels while minimizing hypoglycemia risk.

In the immediate postpartum period, insulin therapy may be discontinued due to the abrupt improvement in insulin sensitivity with the delivery of the placenta and decline in HPL levels. Many newly diagnosed and established T2DM patients may be subsequently managed without insulin, pending their DM duration and beta-cell function, with subsequent pharmacotherapeutic choices pending lactation status.

Gestational Diabetes Mellitus

GDM is traditionally diagnosed by a 100-gram glucose tolerance test following a failed 50-gram glucose screen at 24 weeks. Many patients with GDM are managed successfully with diet and augmented physical activity such as walking. When GDM patients fail to meet glycemic targets of pregnancy, then insulin therapy should be initiated using a regimen similar to patients with pre-existing/newly diagnosed T2DM. Fasting hyperglycemia can be managed with basal insulin and postprandial hyperglycemia can be managed with RAA insulin. In select individuals, basal insulin may be all that is required, and in some individuals only prandial insulin is needed, demonstrating that therapy always needs to be individualized. In the postpartum period, GDM patients by definition are euglycemic because of the abatement of the insulin resistance of pregnancy. These individuals, however, have a 70% lifetime risk of developing T2DM, which is accelerated by the presence of obesity. Patients with a history of GDM need to be counseled on diet, exercise, and weight control to minimize this risk.[11]

Caveat: Not all DM cases that develop during pregnancy are either GDM or new-onset T2DM. Patients may develop true T1DM at any stage during pregnancy.

Hospitalized Patients

T2DM is a common comorbidity in hospitalized patients and can significantly increase the hospital stay and add to morbidity and mortality. Categories of T2DM patients in hospital settings are as follows:

1. Newly discovered T2DM
2. Patients with pre-existing T2DM not requiring insulin therapy prior to admission
3. T2DM patients on insulin therapy prior to admission

Achievement of Glycemic Control

In general, glycemic control will worsen with the augmented insulin resistance of illness, use of glucocorticoids, and the deterioration of beta-cell function from electrolyte disturbances such as hypokalemia. Thus, insulin therapy is frequently needed in the hospitalized patient, depending on the severity of the underlying illness. Metformin should be discontinued in the majority of hospitalized patients due to the augmented risk of lactic acidosis associated with hypoxia, renal insufficiency, and IV contrast studies. Likewise, it would be prudent to discontinue TZDs exenatide, liraglutide and pramlintide in the hospitalized patient; glycemic control can be maintained in the short term with insulin therapy.

Glycemic Goals

The early randomized clinical trials suggested improved outcomes with intensified glycemic control, especially in intensive care unit (ICU) patients.[12,13] For patients in general medical and surgical units, there are no randomized controlled trials to define the goals of glucose control. Tight glycemic control carries the risk of severe hypoglycemia and adverse outcomes, including increased mortality.[14] The inconsistency between studies can be related to different patient selection, glycemic goals, insulin delivery protocols, glucose monitoring frequency, frequency and magnitude of insulin titration, nutritional status, and level of consciousness. A target blood glucose level of 80 to 110 mg/dL in a surgical ICU resulted in reduced morbidity and mortality,[12] whereas the same blood glucose goals in a medical ICU reduced morbidity but not mortality.[13] The frequency of severe hypoglycemic events (blood glucose <40 mg/dL) was six-fold higher in the intensively treated group, and hypoglycemia proved to be an independent risk factor for mortality.

The largest randomized clinical trial was the NICE-SUGAR study, which yielded disappointing results showing increased mortality in critically ill surgical and medical patients with intensive insulin therapy.[14]

Vigilance is needed to avoid hypoglycemia in all patients. Risk factors for hypoglycemia include:

1. Down-titration of corticosteroids
2. Change in the concentration, frequency, rate, and timing of enteral feedings
3. Changes in concentration and/or rate of total parenteral nutrition infusions
4. Missed meals or change in carbohydrate composition of meals
5. Patient physical activity
6. Use of vasopressor agents
7. Changes in endogenous catecholamine levels
8. A change in the insulin infusion rate
9. A change in the insulin to carbohydrate ratio

A consensus statement was published in an effort to make recommendations regarding the best possible glucose control that can be achieved within the constraints of hypoglycemia. The consensus statement made the following recommendation:[15]

1. Critically ill patients in the ICU setting should have a goal blood glucose between 140 and 180 mg/dL, with a tighter goal as low as 110 mg/dL only for selected patients. These goals can be achieved through IV insulin infusion protocols with frequent blood glucose monitoring. Unfortunately, the current CGM systems lack sufficient reliability in the hypoglycemic range to be of benefit in this setting.[16,17]
2. Non-critically ill patients should have a pre-meal glycemic goal of 100 to 140 mg/dL and a random blood glucose goal of <180 mg/dL.

Glycemic Regimens

One of several approaches may be used:

1. In newly diagnosed T2DM patients or in patients with T2DM hitherto not treated with insulin, add basal insulin alone starting at a dose of 10 units/day or 0.2 units/kg of actual body weight. Then use an insulin algorithm for hyperglycemia q4h using RAA or human regular insulin.

2. In patients with T2DM on prior insulin therapy, continue their current basal insulin replacement. Use an algorithm for hyperglycemia q4h with RAA/human regular insulin while NPO. When the patient is able to take PO fluids/food, prandial insulin with RAA can be provided immediately after a meal after assessment of actual carbohydrate intake using the fastest-acting RAA glulisine.

3. Use an insulin drip. There are numerous protocols for insulin drip therapy. Close monitoring of blood glucose is mandatory to achieve glycemic goals and minimize the risk of hypoglycemia. The insulin should be adequately diluted to enable fine-tuning of the infusion rate, especially in leaner, more insulin-sensitive T2DM patients; for example, a dilution of 50 units human regular insulin in 500 cc normal saline gives the ability to titrate in 0.1-unit/hour increments. Drip rates need to be altered promptly should there be any interruption of tube feedings, total parenteral nutrition, and/or the emergence of hypoglycemia or hyperglycemia. Transitioning patients from IV insulin to SC basal-bolus therapy needs to be done cautiously. SC basal insulin needs to be initiated at least 1 hour prior to the discontinuation of the IV insulin, with the basal generally accounting for 50% of the total daily dose.

Caveat: There is no place for using only sliding-scale insulin in the care of the hospitalized patient. Sliding-scale insulin defies normal physiology and is an antiquated and ineffective approach to therapy. Basal insulin must be supplied to control hepatic glucose output and disposal.

References

1. Giovannucci E, Harlan DM, Archer MC, et al. Diabetes and cancer: A consensus report. *Diabetes Care.* 2010;33(7):1674–1685.

2. Johnson JA, Yasmi Y. Glucose-lowering therapies and cancer risk: The trials and tribulations of trials and observations. *Diabetalogia.* 2010;53(9):1823–1826.

3. Pocock SH, Smeeth L. Insulin glargine and malignancy: An unwarranted alarm. *Lancet.* 2009;374(9689):511–513.

4. Monami M, Colombi C, Balzi D, et al. Metformin and cancer occurrence in insulin-treated type 2 diabetic patients. *Diabetes Care.* 2011;34(1):129–131.

5. Peyrot M, Rubin RR, Lauritzen T, et al. on behalf of the International DAWN Advisory Panel. Psychosocial problems and barriers to improved diabetes management: Results of the cross-national Diabetes Attitudes, Wishes and Needs (DAWN) study. *Diab Med.* 2005;22:1379–1385.

6. Gonzalez JS, Safren SA, Cagliero E. Depression, self-care and medication adherence in type 2 diabetes: Relationships across the full range of symptom severity. *Diabetes Care.* 2007;30(9):2222–2227.

7. Young-Hyman DL, Davis CL. Disordered eating behavior in individuals with diabetes: Importance of context, evaluation, and classification. *Diabetes Care.* 2010;33(7):683–689.

8. American Diabetes Association, American Psychiatric Association, American Association of Clinical Endocrinologists, and North American Association for the Study of Obesity Consensus Development Conference on Antipsychotic Drugs, Obesity and Diabetes. *Diabetes Care.* 2004;27(2):596–601.

9. Morrato EH, Newcomer JW, Kamat S. Metabolic screening after the American Diabetes Association's consensus statement on antipsychotic drugs and diabetes. *Diabetes Care.* 2009;32(6):1037–1042.

10. Kitzmiller JL, Block JM, Brown FH, et al. American Diabetes Association Consensus Statement for Managing pre-existing diabetes for pregnancy: Summary of evidence and consensus recommendations for care. *Diabetes Care.* 2008;31(5):1060–1079.

11. Landon MB, Spong CY, Thom E, et al. A multicenter, randomized trial of treatment for mild gestational diabetes. *N Engl J Med.* 2009;361(14):1339–1348.

12. Van den Bergh G, Wouters D, Weekers F, et al. Intensive insulin therapy in critically ill patients. *N Engl J Med.* 2001;345(19):1359–1367.

13. Van den Bergh G, Wilmer A, Hermans G, et al. Intensive insulin therapy in the medical ICU. *N Engl J Med.* 2006;354(5):449–461.

14. The NICE-SUGAR Study Investigators. Intensive versus conventional glucose control in critically ill patients. *N Engl J Med.* 2009;360(13):1283–1297.

15. Moghissi ES, Korytkowski MT, DiNardo M, et al. American College of Endocrinology and American Diabetes Association consensus statement on inpatient diabetes and glycemic control. *Endocr Pract.* 2006;12(4):458–468.

16. Goldberg PA, Siegel MD, Russell RR, et al. Experience with the continuous glucose monitoring system in a medical intensive care unit. *Diabetes Technol Ther.* 2004;6(3):339–347.

17. Murakam A, Gutierrez MA, Lage SH, et al. A continuous glucose monitoring system in critical care patients in the intensive care unit. *Comput Cardio.* 2006;33(17–20 Sept):223–236.

Chapter 9

Prevention of T2DM

Type 2 DM

The Diabetes Prevention Program (DPP)[1] clearly showed that a 58% relative risk reduction for developing T2DM at the IGT stage was possible with a program of diet and exercise. Similar results were achieved in Scandinavian trials, confirming the DPP findings.[2] Pharmacotherapy with metformin in the DPP yielded a 31% relative risk reduction. The combination of metformin and TLC was not studied in the DPP but does hold promise for synergistic effects. TZD therapy has been shown to reduce the rate of development of T2DM, especially as evidenced in the DREAM (Diabetes Reduction Assessment with Ramipril and Rosiglitazone Medication) trial, in which there was a 62% relative risk reduction for development of T2DM at the stage of IGT, with >50% of the patients reverting to normoglycemia.[3] The STOP-NIDDM (Study to Prevent Non-Insulin-Dependent Diabetes Mellitus) trial, which used the α-glucosidase inhibitor acarbose, showed a 25% relative risk reduction for the development of T2DM at the stage of IGT. The STOP-NIDDM trial also demonstrated a 49% relative risk reduction for cardiovascular events.[4]

Currently there is no FDA-approved pharmacotherapy for IGT or isolated IFG, so the use of any of these aforementioned agents would be considered off-label. Additionally, there is some debate whether any of the available pharmacotherapies actually prevent T2DM versus delay the onset of T2DM. In general, when pharmacotherapy is stopped, the glucose tolerance deteriorates.

Prevention strategies should be considered in high-risk populations, such as patients with:

1. IGT/IFG
2. History of prior GDM
3. Strong positive family history of early-onset T2DM
4. Obesity, especially in the setting of a high waist:hip ratio
5. Essential HTN
6. Elevated serum triglycerides and low HDL-C
7. Hyperuricemia and history of gout
8. PCOS

Obesity

Obesity starts in childhood for many individuals, so lifestyle modification must start at a young age in the home and the school. Parents and teachers, not to mention health care professionals, should serve as role models in this regard.

Community outreach programs have been established to combat both obesity and T2DM. These have been conducted through schools, churches, community centers, and even employers. Improvement in school nutrition is a major target of obesity reduction. Larger employers sometimes foster fitness and weight control via onsite fitness centers, subsidized gym memberships, and healthier food options in office cafeterias. The results of the Flerbaix Laventie Ville Santé (FLVS) study in France is grounds for optimism. In that community-based study, lifestyle intervention revolving around diet and exercise reduced the prevalence of overweight children from 17.8% to 8.8%.[5]

References

1. Diabetes Prevention Program Research Group. Reduction in the incidence of type 2 diabetes with lifestyle intervention or metformin. *N Engl J Med.* 2002;346(6):393–403.

2. Tuomilheto J, Lindstrom J, Eriksson JG, et al. for the Finnish Diabetes Prevention Group. Prevention of type 2 diabetes mellitus by changes in lifestyle among subjects with impaired glucose tolerance. *N Engl J Med.* 2001;344(18):1343–1350.

3. The DREAM (Diabetes Reduction Assessment with Ramipril and Rosiglitazone Medication) Trial Investigators. Effect of rosiglitazone on the frequency of diabetes in patients with impaired glucose tolerance or impaired fasting glucose: A randomized controlled trial. *Lancet.* 2006;368(9541):1096–1105.

4. Chiasson J-L, Josse RF, Gomis R, et al. Acarbose for prevention of type 2 diabetes mellitus: The STOP-NIDDM randomized trial. *Lancet.* 2002;359(9323):2072–2077.

5. Romon M, Lommez A, Tafflet M, et al. Downward trends in the prevalence of childhood overweight in the setting of 12-year school- and community-based programmes. *Public Health Nutrition.* 2009;12(10):1735–1741.

Conclusion

Intensive diabetes management from the time of diagnosis yields microvascular and macrovascular risk reduction. Therapeutic lifestyle changes need to be advocated from the start. Practitioners need to avoid clinical inertia and advance pharmacotherapy promptly as beta-cell function declines. Failure to optimize glycemic control early in the course of T2DM appears to result in a "legacy effect" that is not readily reversible. Diabetes is clearly a serious disease that warrants early diagnosis and intensive treatment of all risk factors, including lifestyle, hypertension, and lipids, from the outset to prevent devastating and costly microvascular and macrovascular complications.

Index